THE END OF MIGRAINES

150 WAYS TO STOP YOUR PAIN

ALEXANDER MAUSKOP, MD

Advance praise

"I enjoyed reading this book which is intended as a comprehensive but practical resource for persons with migraines. The text is thorough but very readable. Dr. Mauskop employs his extensive clinical experience with historical anecdotes, scientific references and a dash of humor. He covers a wide range of options for those with migraine ranging from non-pharmacologic treatments (avoidance of triggers, healthy lifestyle, physical measures, behavioral measures and even neuro-modulation) to supplements and the whole range of acute and preventive non-prescription and prescription remedies. This text includes links to put the reader in touch with resources mentioned in the book through the internet including scientific references and videos demonstrating various techniques. It includes information about other types of headaches which may be confused with migraine and when to seek medical advice. Dr. Mauskop's practical approach to dealing with migraine is exemplified by using evidence-based medicine when possible and relying on his extensive clinical experience when there is less evidence. Throughout the book, common sense prevails. As a "person with migraine" I found the book informative and a resource that I would read in its entirety but then keep as a reference. The cost is quite low which should make it very accessible to anyone wishing to become well-informed about this very prevalent but misunderstood condition."

Thomas N. Ward, MD
Emeritus Professor of Neurology, Dartmouth Geisel School of Medicine
Editor-in-Chief, *Headache: The Journal of Head and Face Pain*

■ ■ ■

"*The End of Migraines: 150 ways to stop your pain* by Alexander Mauskop, is a remarkable book, and brings something new to the library of headache resources for patients. Dr. Mauskop, a longtime advocate for non-medicinal treatments for headaches, covers every imaginable option here from supplements to herbal treatments to many lifestyle and behavioral strategies. But he draws on his solid academic background (he is a professor and researcher) to also enumerate the pharmaceutical and device treatment options as well. And based on his extensive experience in treating thousands of people with migraine, he rates each of the treatment choices contained in this book as more or less likely to be useful.

As he explains in the wonderfully written introductory section of the book, Dr. Mauskop's approach is not always based on evidence, but rather it is designed to fill gaps where evidence is lacking. The reader finds a world of options for reducing the burden of migraine, and as a result, regains hope.

The writing style is clear and concise, and readers will have the sense that they are sitting with Dr. Mauskop and hearing his advice first hand. The hyperlinks throughout the text expand options for delving more deeply into many topics. This is a highly readable and practical guide which will be valuable to all people battling migraine, as well as their family and friends."

Morris Levin, MD, Professor of Neurology
Director of the Headache Center at UCSF Medical Center

■ ■ ■

"Knowledge is power and migraine patients will be empowered with knowledge after reading *The End of Migraines*. A leading authority shares his decades of clinical experience on the nuances of migraine care, from the standard medical approaches to acupuncture, behavioral, dietary and other approaches to prevent or treat migraine. Not only will migraineurs benefit from this book, but so will neurologists!"

Orrin Devinsky, MD

Professor of Neurology, Neurosurgery, and Psychiatry, NYU Grossman School of Medicine

■ ■ ■

"Dr. Mauskop has treated thousands of patients with migraine during decades of clinical experience. He is a gifted educator and this volume showcases his extraordinary ability to condense evidence and clinical observation into pithy analysis and practical suggestions. His goal is to describe and evaluate the immense amount of information available about the diverse strategies—self-management, behavioral, and medical—that have been shown to impact the occurrence and treatment of migraine. The work will be empowering for those who suffer with this malady and will provide a foundation for lifestyle decisions and discussions with health professions about migraine therapy."

Russell K. Portenoy, MD

Professor of Neurology and Family and Social Medicine
Albert Einstein College of Medicine

■ ■ ■

"As someone who suffers from migraine, and as a practicing neurologist, I am aware of the disruptive and painful beast that can interfere with work, leisure, and just plain life. For quite some time, I have been looking for a migraine manual that is comprehensive yet easy to read, simple to navigate, timely, and inexpensive. Dr. Alexander Mauskop, MD, FAAN, an internationally renowned expert in the field, has written just such a treatise. And I am not at all surprised. This e-book will be of immeasurable help to my fellow migraine sufferers."

Michael Rubin, MD, FRCP(C), FAAN
Professor of Clinical Neurology
Weill Cornell Medicine

■ ■ ■

"In this practical guide to the practice of migraine, Dr. Mauskop is providing a most comprehensive reference to the essence and the treatment of migraine. He touches everything – from music to food, sleep to herbs, drugs and devices that might do good to migraine sufferers. His hyperlinks make the book an easy base to further exploration of the field, and his frequent visits to relevant cultural vignettes makes the reading enjoyable. The book it meant mainly to serve patients who want to know more about their migraine; is their headache really migraine, what can they do about it in lifestyle changes, what are the non-pharmacological treatments, alternative treatments and what is the current state of the pharmacological approaches to treat and prevent migraine. The interested patient will be able to better know the treatment he or she is receiving, what to expect as far as efficacy and side effects, and what are the alternatives in case treatment proves not suitable. This is an era of free internet searches that many patients perform, often leading to an unbalanced picture of the clinical situation, emphasizing the more severe sides, yielding higher stress and sometimes hindering the therapeutic effects. It is important to have a balanced reference, that gives a uniform frame to all treatments, and allows a sound assessment for the non-professional reader. The latter can use the ratings given by the author, using his rich experience, of the various treatments, as a general guide to efficacy. Given the comprehensiveness of the text, I believe health care professionals can also enjoy the book as a handy reference for various details in the management of migraine."

David Yarnitsky, MD
Professor, Rappaport Faculty of Medicine of the Technion-Israel Institute of Technology, Israel
Director, Department of Neurology, Rambam Health Care Campus

■ ■ ■

"Dr. Mauskop, a highly experienced specialist in headache medicine, has compiled a book which will answer many of the questions that those with migraine frequently ask. This is particularly timely given the multiple new treatments and approaches to the management of those with migraine. He discusses medications, non-medication treatments, and triggers of attacks. Those suffering from migraine, or those having someone close to them suffering from migraine, would be wise to read this information and incorporate this information into their own management plan."

Mark W. Green MD, FAAN
Director of Headache and Pain Medicine
Professor of Neurology, Anesthesiology, and Rehabilitation Medicine
Icahn School of Medicine at Mount Sinai

■ ■ ■

"One of the pitfalls of the world wide web is that you can find a tremendous amount of information but you cannot be sure if the information is correct. Therefore, you need experienced commentators to help you to find your own way through the jungle. This is especially true in the case of migraine. Migraine is not only the most prevalent neurological disorder but also one of the most complex ones, since migraine has many points of contact with a whole range of other disorders (e.g. cardio- and cerebrovascular disorders, anxiety disorders, depression, restless legs syndrome, inflammatory bowel disease, epilepsy, Tourette syndrome, neurodermatitis and many more). Another important point in the planning and later evaluation of the success of therapy is that, as in nearly all medical treatments, in migraine we also have to consider a treatment-specific effect and an unspecific, context-dependent treatment effect, which, even in the therapy with monoclonal antibodies, accounts for about 2/3 of the observed effect. Therefore, it is clear that an approach like "one therapy fits all patients" cannot be the answer. The book by Alexander Mauskop bridges this gap and gives the interested patient seeking personal solutions a short overview of the factors which could influence his or her migraine. This enables patients to select their own interventions. In other words, the book allows the patient to become an informed partner of the doctor."

Andreas Straube, MD
Professor of Neurology and Clinical Neurophysiology
Head of the Upper Bavarian Headache Center
Munich, Germany

■ ■ ■

"Because of their debilitating nature and high prevalence in the population, migraine headaches are too important to leave exclusively to physicians. Similarly to the condition which I, as an endocrinologist, manage on a daily basis – namely, diabetes – migraines require astute awareness of lifestyle factors and active participation by the patient. This is why the monograph by Dr. Alexander Mauskop, Director of New York Headache Center and Professor of Clinical Neurology at SUNY Downstate Medical Center, is an invaluable tool for both physicians and patients who deal with migraine.

The book covers environmental influences, lifestyle measures (e.g. food, and exercise), complementary methods of treatment (e.g. acupuncture, music, Thai Chi, herbal products) as well as Food and Drug Administration approved pharmaceuticals. The volume is written clearly and is fun to read.

I recommend *The End of Migraines* with immense enthusiasm to both patients and health care professionals whose life is impacted by migraine. This monograph is certain to dramatically improve the quality of life of all those affected by this important condition whose management requires a holistic multidisciplinary approach."

Leonid Poretsky, MD

Professor of Medicine, Donald and Barbara Zucker School of Medicine at Hofstra/Northwell
Director of Medicine – Endocrinology/Metabolism, Lenox Hill Hospital

■ ■ ■

"This comprehensive and engaging book by a well-known headache neurologist with decades of experience is a must-read reference for anyone living with migraines. It provides an exploration and explanation of a broad range of conventional and non-traditional treatment options in an easy-to-use format. In an age where migraineurs are increasingly educated about their condition and active participants in their management, this book provides up-to-date information on an extensive array of topics and therapies, allowing patients to navigate the treatment landscape in a way that best suits their individual circumstances."

Christina Sun-Edelstein, MD, FRACP

Senior Lecturer, University of Melbourne
Headache Clinic at St. Vincent's Hospital, Melbourne

■ ■ ■

"Dr. Alex Mauskop is that unusual physician, a man who is willing to consider all types of therapies and to review evidence for these treatments. He is open-minded, and his book *The End of Migraines: 150 ways to stop your pain*, is a fascinating look at a large number of potential approaches to treating migraine. Dr. Mauskop lists many approaches, some clearly established as effective, some worth considering for future research, and he describes what is known about these therapies and what is not. He writes in a manner that is clear and helpful, and those with migraine will be interested in his take on a large number of potential treatments for migraine."

Stewart J. Tepper, MD

Professor of Neurology
Geisel School of Medicine at Dartmouth

■ ■ ■

"This is a remarkably readable and comprehensive overview of Headache Medicine. Dr Mauskop is an experienced clinician who manages to seamlessly integrate the best evidence along with practical insights throughout the headache terrain. I highly recommend this book to health care professionals as well as the general public."

Steven M. Baskin, PhD
Director of Behavioral Medicine
New England Institute for Neurology and Headache

■ ■ ■

"Dr. Mauskop shares a lifetime of his clinical passions, experience, and work in an easy to read book on combating headaches that patients suffer from every day. For those that don't have the opportunity to have direct patient care by Dr. Mauskop, here is the chance to inform and empower yourself, share with your care team, and start on the path to wellbeing and less headache disability. This book shares the opportunity for identifying the diagnosis and differentiating migraine-like headaches, 150+ treatments of headache including preventative and treatment medications, and guidance on when the headaches are an emergency. I commend Dr. Mauskop on sharing his wisdom with a large population of headache sufferers and treaters."

Neel Mehta, MD
Medical Director of Pain Medicine at the Weill-Cornell Pain Medicine Center and New York-Presbyterian Hospital

■ ■ ■

"I highly recommend this book for those struggling to find a solution to their head pain. With the wide range of approaches available, having a sound reference guide such as this is gold! With Dr. Mauskop's 30 years in practice and openness to both pharmaceutical and non-pharmaceutical tools, this is one of the best books to date on this subject matter. Topics range from testing and diary keeping to supplements, lifestyle techniques and/or pharmaceuticals with the goal of meeting patients where they are to achieve optimal outcomes. A must read!"

Trupti Gokani, MD
Board Certified Neurologist/Ayurvedic Counselor and NLP Coach
Author of *The Mysterious Mind: How to Use Ancient Wisdom and Modern Science to Heal Your Headaches and Reclaim Your Health*

■ ■ ■

"Dr. Mauskop's newest book encompasses evidence-based headache medicine for both patients and physicians like myself. This book, *The End of Migraines: 150 ways to stop your pain* is a comprehensive guide which can be used to guide treatment based on the preferences of the person with migraine. I really enjoyed the section on non-drug approaches because many of my patients specifically ask for treatment approaches such as acupuncture, diet modification and supplements. I also really like the message to patients and providers that there are a plethora of treatment approaches for migraine and so there is always something different we can turn to."

Deena Kuruvilla, MD
Neurologist and Headache Specialist
Yale School of Medicine

■ ■ ■

"The reputable and celebrated neurologist from New York, Dr. Alexander Mauskop, in his newest book *The End of Migraines: 150 ways to stop your pain*, describes a thorough and competent approach of Migraine and headache. Bouncing without restrictions from one topic to another, from the clinical presentation to orient sufferers and colleagues to the upcoming and emerging therapies, from the importance of keeping a headache diary to the circumstances when you have to be tested, he describes and approaches the spectrum of migraine in a way everyone should listen. In addition, the book examines the recently approved anti-CGRP treatments either for the treatment of migraine as a disease as well as the gepants and ditans for headache attacks. In a time of media campaigns regarding new treatments, patients may be confused and create unrealistic expectations. This book clarifies this issue and presents reasonable points that should be useful. After 35 years of dealing with migraine sufferers, I may say that this book encompasses nearly everything one should know. It is, for sure, a must-read project from an accomplished professional with many years of dedication and experience in headache medicine and migraine."

Abouch Krymchantowski, MD, MSc, PhD, FAAH
Director and Founder of Headache Center of Rio, Brazil

■ ■ ■

"In this book written by a well-respected headache specialist, you will be able to find quick but detailed answers to all the doubts you can imagine on migraine treatments".

Julio Pascual Gomez, MD, PhD
Professor of Medicine of the University of Cantabria
Director of Neurology at the University Hospital Marqués de Valdecilla, Spain.

■ ■ ■

"This is an excellent, must-read book for anyone who suffers from chronic headaches. It is full of clinical pearls that even neurologists and specialists will find most helpful."

Gayatri Devi, MD, MS, FAAN

Director of *Park Avenue Neurology*
Clinical Professor of Neurology at *SUNY Downstate*
Attending Neurologist at *Lenox Hill Hospital*

■ ■ ■

"Once again, Alex Mauskop has delivered a lucid and lively overview of the causes, consequences, and management of that uniquely human problem...that of headache."

Richard Lechtenberg, MD

The author of *Synopsis of Neurology, Disorders of the Cerebellum, The Diagnosis and Treatment of Epilepsy,* and other books.

■ ■ ■

"Dr. Mauskop and I have known each other for decades. I learned something about him that I have never known in reading his book. He and I are both migraine patients. His migraines assuredly are not the same as mine or vice versa, which is one of the essential points from this book. From our conversations, I know that we don't share the same beliefs in every treatment that is available for patients. This is because we, too, bring different strengths, abilities, and experience to our patients. Everyone who has migraines is unique and will respond to treatments differently, and likely we will find that this is due to our specific genetics. Of all that Dr.Mauskop has done over the years, what makes him unique is this. A noted journalist once said that a good doctor treats diseases. A great doctor treats patients. I consider him to be a great doctor. He takes each individual for what they are and the nature of their headaches for what it is. He takes a wide-open search for the best approaches to help that patient. Not the next one or the one before. He knows the research that has been done over time to ascertain the nature of migraine and other headaches. He has studied the therapeutic options and their potential for not just success but also patient safety.

In some respects, patients are their own best doctors. They have their ideas about the nature of their headaches and experience in trying to manage them. They come to physicians like Dr. Mauskop and me because we can not only prescribe treatments they otherwise would not have access to, but we have decades of or and research and experience in working with many thousands of patients. This allows headache medicine specialists to bring a greater level of expertise to the patient and afford them options that they can consider on their merit and potential to help them control their migraine and other headache disorders.

Sadly, many persons have little if any concept of what it means to have a migraine and other disabling headache disorders. To many, they think that if two aspirin is good enough to control their headaches that they should be good enough to control yours. Only in the past few decades has there been substantial recognition by physicians of the nature and impact of headache. Our medical education system has not kept pace with the myriad of developments that have occurred, and too few physicians receive anything passing for adequate training in headache medicine. This all too often leaves patients in a sad situation of not finding success on their own and not finding it with the family physician.

This book won't make you an expert in headaches, but it will increase your knowledge about headaches and their varied treatments. It will make you a better patient for your provider, one who is informed and open to exploring options. Options that sometimes require a lot of you, others that will require taking medications or bearing costs of treatments when you would rather not. I love going "toe to toe" with my patients. Why? I know they are committed to their treatment and getting well. That makes me all the more determined to do everything I can to help them in their quest. This book is just one more example of how Dr. Mauskop has undertaken this challenge, which extends well beyond the exam and waiting room to all those who bear the price of challenging headaches. It offers the potential to gain control of your headaches and have a life in your hands, not those of your headache disorder dictating your vitality and well being. "

Frederick G. Freitag, DO FAHS
Professor of Neurology
Medical College of Wisconsin

■ ■ ■

"This book, by the noted founder and director of the New York Headache Center, is so chock full of useful information that the reader may be surprised to learn it is packed into less than 200 concise pages. Unlike his prior three texts, *The End of Migraines: 150 ways to stop your pain* is an ebook, which provides the dual advantages of lower cost ($3.95) and the presence of many valuable hyperlinks. A print format is also available. Dr. Mauskop derived much of the content from his more than 800 blog posts over fifteen years, along with reader comments.

Dr. Mauskop, himself a migraine sufferer, wields a compassionate and at times playful touch with his prose, with literary quotes sprinkled throughout, invoking other neurologist-writers such as Edward Liveing and Oliver Sacks. The book covers a plethora of migraine treatments, from rigorously studied pharmaceuticals to vitamins and supplements to hands-on techniques such as acupuncture and Feldenkrais – each ranked (on a zero to ten scale) to give the reader meaningful context on which of the 150 treatments may be better starting points as they begin their migraine treatment journey.

The End of Migraines: 150 ways to stop your pain is a must-read not only for migraine sufferers but should be a required text for all health care practitioners who treat them."

Peter McAllister, MD, FAAN

Medical Director, New England Institute for Neurology and Headache
Chief Medical Officer, New England Institute for Clinical Research

■ ■ ■

"Dr. Alex Mauskop is my go-to physician for patients with difficult migraines. *The End of Migraines* is a distillation of his wisdom and experience, a comprehensive, wholistic self-help guide for headaches. If you suffer from headaches or have been told you have migraine, this is the first book you should read."

Leo Galland, MD

Author, *The Allergy Solution*

■ ■ ■

The End of Migraines: 150 ways to stop your pain

Copyright 2021, by Alexander Mauskop

ISBN: 978-1-7362868-0-7 (Paperback edition)

ISBN: 978-1-7362868-1-4 (eBook edition)

www.NYHeadache.com

New York Headache Center

Dedication

For Karen, my wife and best friend

Acknowledgments

I am indebted to all my patients who entrusted me with their care.

I am grateful to my colleagues who took the time to read and recommend this book.

Thank you to my friend, Robin Flicker, who helped edit this book.

Table of Contents

Foreword

The recent advances in our understanding and management of migraine have collided with the exponential growth of electronic communication to produce a tremendous volume of related information. So great is that volume, so broad the range of issues addressed and so diverse the multitude of sources that even the migraine-savvy may find it difficult to access reliable information relevant to their needs. Thus arises again the great dilemma of the Age of Electronic Information: while it may be helpful to have a sizable haystack, how can we find therein the needles of information we seek? And, if found, can that information be trusted?

Happily, at least for individuals with migraine who are dismayed by the existing haystack of relevant information, in his new book entitled *The End of Migraines* Dr. Alexander Mauskop has greatly simplified the task. In only 8 well-organized chapters, with writing that is clear, concise and easily comprehended, Dr. Mauskop guides the reader through the full spectrum of migraine; his emphasis is on therapeutic management, both pharmacologic and non-pharmacologic, but blended with this are helpful insights on topics ranging from the identification of migraine triggers to the question of when diagnostic testing may be indicated; he even finds time to delve into special circumstances such as menstrual migraine and a description of other headache disorders which may be mistaken for migraine.

In its range and clarity, this book nicely reflects its author. A gifted clinician, scientist and educator, Dr. Mauskop has worked for many years to raise the standard of care for migraine and has made important contributions to the arsenal of evidence-based migraine therapies. At the same time, he has maintained a pragmatic, open-minded approach to the practice of headache medicine which embraces the truism that an absence of evidence does not necessarily foretell an absence of benefit. He has been a pioneer in the exploration of what he characterizes in this book as "non-drug approaches"; these include the use of supplements such as magnesium, a treatment intervention he championed long before it became widely used by medical providers everywhere.

1

In describing a wide variety of therapies for the reader, Dr. Mauskop is careful to distinguish between those which possess a solid foundation of scientific evidence and those which do not. Given his extensive clinical experience, his deep knowledge of migraine and his clear-eyed approach to the evaluation of migraine therapies, I particularly appreciated his having graded many of the therapies he describes on a personal "1-10" scale. I know of few other headache subspecialists whose personal opinion of a given therapy I would trust as much.

Highly appropriate for migraine, an extraordinarily common medical disorder whose biologic and therapeutic landscape is ever-evolving, ***The End of Migraines*** is published in electronic form. As such, it will be both readily available to that 12% of the general population actively afflicted with the disorder and also easily updated as new information accumulates.

Dr. Mauskop's comprehensive, accessible and dynamic manual for understanding and managing migraine is a *tour de force*.

John F. Rothrock, MD
Professor of Neurology, The George Washington University School of Medicine

Preface

Trying to keep up with health advice can feel like surfing the Net for weather forecasts: what you find is always changing, often contradictory and rarely encouraging.

—*Julian Baggini*

I ndeed, medical advice is always changing. For that reason, I decided on the eBook format to be able to update this book regularly, as new scientific data emerges.

Some of the advice in this book may seem contradictory. Snacking helps, but so does losing weight; caffeine is good and caffeine is bad; exercise prevents migraines, but it can also trigger them; avoid drugs, except when you can't; and so on. The reason for these seeming contradictions is that no one approach works for everyone. What alleviates one person's migraine may worsen another's. If you can't obtain relief on your own, or need a prescription for a drug that is not over the counter, by all means, see a doctor or a nurse practitioner.

Another reason I settled on an eBook format is to make it more affordable. If you prefer to read on paper, you can have the book printed by Kindle Publishing. You will not be able to access the hyperlinks, but those are not essential. The electronic format allows you to increase the font size to reduce strain on your eyes, a common problem in people with migraines.

The book is short enough to read through in a couple of hours. If you are interested in more information, there are numerous hyperlinks that will lead you to the description of scientific studies, supplements, gadgets, and drugs you may be interested in trying.

Many of the entries in this book are adapted from my blog, nyheadache.com/blog. There are nearly 800 posts written between 2007 until mid-2020, and several thousand comments from readers. I decided to write this

3

book because many people commented that the information on the blog was useful to them.

I hope that the description of more than 150 options will be encouraging.

Introduction

I have tried, in this book, to distill over 30 years of experience treating migraine patients. Having migraines myself gave me additional insights and enables me to say that I truly feel your pain. However, everyone's experience is unique, and my pain is not exactly your pain. My migraines have never interfered with my life, although I've had periods of daily migraines that lasted for years. My migraines have continued to respond quickly, completely, and without side effects to sumatriptan tablets or injections. Twice, I've given myself injections of Botox and an infusion of magnesium. I have tried injections and tablets of several drugs and various supplements. What made the biggest difference for me is when I started to meditate for 30 minutes every day and exercise at least three times a week. My major triggers are alcohol and lack of sleep. Avoiding those has helped as well.

You and I are in good company. Elie Wiesel, Lewis Carroll, Serena Williams, Kareem Abdul Jabbar, Elizabeth Taylor, Kanye West, Friedrich Nietzche, Napoleon, Charles Darwin, Thomas Jefferson, Miguel de Cervantes, Sigmund Freud, John F. Kennedy, Julius Caesar, half of all neurologists, and two-thirds of headache specialists suffer from migraine.

If many remedies are prescribed for an illness, you may be certain that the illness has no cure.

—Anton Chekhov, Cherry Orchard

Chekhov was not only a writer but also a physician. Migraine is an excellent example of his remark about illnesses with many remedies and no current cure. The good news is that a true cure is likely to come when genetic engineering becomes commonplace. This may take a decade or two.

How, then, can I pronounce *The End of Migraines?* Because even though you may remain predisposed to getting migraines, this book tells you how to stop having them. You may still be at risk, but if migraines occur a few times a year or less, if you learn how to prevent or stop them, it is as good as a cure.

Another encouraging feature of this condition is that as people get older, two out of three stop having migraine. How old do you have to be for it to go away? In women, it often happens after menopause. In men, migraines often stop in their 50's and 60's. Migraine attacks sometimes stop for no apparent reason.

The main message of this book is that migraine doesn't have to run or ruin your life. You can regain control and stop your suffering. You will not need all 150 or even 50 treatments described here. However, having 150 options means that there is an excellent chance of finding the ones that work for you.

Many patients have implored me, *please do not give up on me like my last neurologist who said that there is nothing else that he could do for me*. It is not acceptable for a patient to be shamed or made to feel that they have "failed" when a treatment doesn't work. You may want to try to find doctors who don't blame you for failing to respond to the prescribed treatments. And for doctors reading this book, please never dismiss patients for not getting better under your care and continue to search for a solution.

Evidence-based medicine is not enough

I love the statement by British mycologist, Merlin Sheldrake in his book on fungi, *Entangled Life: How Fungi Make Our Worlds, Change Our Minds and Shape our Futures*: "Science isn't an exercise in cold-blooded rationality. Scientists are – and have always been – emotional, creative, intuitive, whole human beings, asking questions about a world that was never made to be catalogued and systematized."

This is true in medicine. Trying to treat every patient strictly according to evidence-based guidelines is misguided.

Evidence-based medicine (EBM) is defined as a conscientious, explicit, judicious, and reasonable use of modern, best evidence in making decisions about the care of individual patients. Throughout this book and in practice, I've tried to adhere to the goals of EBM. You can find many links to scientific articles that support various treatments. When a link to a scientific study is provided, you need not assume that the study proves something. Much of the time, studies offer merely observations and case reports. Though valuable, they are not definitive, but rather suggestions for further observations and study. Rigorously scientific studies have inherent flaws. In a study that involves hundreds of patients, each patient will have a different genetic makeup, diet and activity level, psychological profile, and many other variables. We know for certain that migraine is not the same even in members of the same family. Another limitation of EBM is that it is simplistic. It fails to take into account the complexity of doctor-patient interactions. In the words of an Australian ethicist, Dr. Narcyz Ghinea, it presumes "that physicians cannot be trusted to utilize their extensive training and skills to make reasonable decisions in the best interests of their patients."

150+ treatments

Many of the treatment ideas that I describe in this book are not just off-label (that is, not approved by the FDA) but may appear to be off-the-wall. Over the years, I've continued to look for unorthodox approaches out of necessity. Some doctors limit their treatment to the few drugs that the FDA has approved for migraines. If those drugs don't work, or if they cause troublesome side effects, many doctors will wash their hands and tell the patient that there are no other options. I am not such a doctor, and I encourage you to seek out doctors who do not dismiss your suffering simply because you do not respond to traditional treatment modalities. Time and again, I see people who have "tried everything," yet found no relief. Because doctors don't like to fail, they often unwittingly send a message that the patient has failed. This is never true, and if this book does anything, I hope it emboldens you to keep seeking relief, not to give up on or blame yourself for the pain you experience from migraine.

I believe that if a treatment is safe, inexpensive, and has been reported to help, it may be worth trying, even if it has not been subjected to rigorous clinical trials. Sometimes these treatments work not because they are truly effective, but because of the placebo response or because the disease of migraine has resolved on its own. Finding relief is what matters. How it happened matters less. Unlike a controlled clinical trial, the practice of medicine is more art than science.

Although medications can be lifesavers, you may be able to avoid them. Of the 150 treatments, non-drug therapies take up significantly more than half of the pages in this book.

About supplements and medications

Each supplement mentioned in the book has a hyperlink to its description on the website of the National Center for Complementary and Integrative

Health (part of the National Institutes of Health), on WebMD, or on the Integrative Medicine part of the website of Memorial Sloan-Kettering Cancer Center (where I did my Pain Fellowship in the Department of Neurology from 1984 to 1986).

Medications are referred to by their generic names. Common brand names are listed in parentheses and are capitalized. Most drugs listed in this book are not approved by the FDA (or its European equivalent, European Medicines Agency) specifically for the treatment of migraine headaches. Those that are, I have marked with an asterisk. An asterisk also marks several stimulation devices that were cleared to treat migraine headaches. Most drugs have a brief description of their utility in treating migraines, important side effects, and other facts. If you are interested in more details, click on the hyperlink included for each drug. The link will take you to MedlinePlus, "an online health information resource for patients and their families and friends". This is a trustworthy source of information compiled by the United States National Library of Medicine, though it often overwhelms with information. It will seem to you that most drugs have many potentially dangerous side effects. The risk of these side effects is real, which is why drugs should be avoided when possible. The first half of this book advances non-drug approaches. However, drugs are often necessary and can be life-changing. Along with a healthcare provider, one should always weigh the pros and cons.

To make such decisions a little easier, I gave every drug and some of the non-drug treatments a grade. The grade is on a scale of 1 to 10, taking into account efficacy, safety, sometimes cost, convenience, and my overall impression. The grade is subjective, but it is based on my experience treating thousands of patients. I did not include any drugs that I would give a grade as low as 1, and no treatment earns a grade of 10. This doesn't mean that some drugs for some patients cannot earn a top grade; as mentioned earlier, each person is unique so that no drug is perfect for all people all the time. At the end of the book, I provide my top 10 list of treatments.

Is it worth trying a treatment that I assign a rating of 2 or 3? It depends. An herbal remedy, a vitamin supplement, or an electrical stimulation device may be effective for only one out of three or four people. Little is lost by trying these low-rated treatments if traditional approaches do not work, cause side effects, or you are just afraid of potential side effects.

You may respond to a low-rated drug or treatment because of your unique genetic makeup, different ways that your brain is wired, different ways that your body reacts to stress, environment, food, or drugs.

There is no right or wrong way to go about trying any of the 150 treatments. You may want to look through all the options listed and try a few at a time. Trying to do 10 things at the same time is difficult. But if you try only one approach at a time, you may not find a solution for a long time. If you want to find a solution faster, it makes sense to try a few treatments at a time. How will you know which one helped? It's simple. First, get your headaches under control. Once you do, it will be easy to figure out which treatment was responsible. Start dropping them one at a time. Just don't drop exercise, meditation, a healthy diet, and good sleeping habits. It is also possible that each ingredient contributes perhaps, 10-20% to the improvement. By combining them, you may end up with 80% or even 100% of relief.

It makes more sense to combine treatments of different types, rather than take three different drugs or five different herbal products. Here is an example of a useful protocol: a healthy diet, exercise, meditation, magnesium for prevention, and, when a migraine strikes, a prescription drug such as sumatriptan. Another scenario: stop caffeine if you are overdoing it, reduce sugar intake, exercise, meditate, and take an herbal supplement, boswellia. For an acute attack, take ibuprofen. If non-drug approaches alone do not sufficiently reduce the frequency of attacks, try a daily medicine, Botox injections, or one of the CGRP monoclonal antibodies for prevention.

Find a coach, a partner, or a sympathetic friend

Having a partner or a coach can help you stay motivated to keep looking for a solution and to adhere to a particular treatment long enough to see results. This could be your spouse, a close friend, a health coach (health coaching is a growing field), a nurse-practitioner, or a psychotherapist.

Having frequent migraines is bad enough, but a lack of understanding from family, friends, and colleagues makes living with migraines so much worse. In the introduction to the first edition of his now-classic textbook on headaches published in 1969, Australian neurologist James Lance describes the attitude of family members, friends, co-workers, and many physicians: "It is easy for a person who has never been troubled with headaches to lose patience with those who are plagued by them. The reaction of the virtuous observer may pass through a phase of sympathetic concern to one of frustrated tolerance and, finally, to a mood of irritation and resentment in which the recurrence of headaches is attributed to a defective personality or escape from unpleasant life situations."

If you feel that your friends and relatives don't take your migraines seriously, you can try to educate them, bring them to doctor visits, or engage in family therapy. This is not easy but can help you gain support while you are exploring treatments listed in this book. Your coach could also benefit from a technique called <u>LEAP that was first developed by a psychologist, Dr. Xavier Amador</u> for families of people with mental illness. It can be adapted for chronic migraines. LEAP stands for listen, empathize, agree (or accept), and partner.

One of the most vivid, poetic descriptions of a migraine experience I've come across is in the novel *Atonement*, by Ian McEwan:

"...Emily Tallis had withdrawn from the white glare of the afternoon's heat to a cool and darkened bedroom. She was not in pain, not yet, but she was retreating before its threat. There were illuminated points in her vision, little pinpricks, as though the worn fabric of the visible world was being held up against a far brighter light. She felt in the top right corner of her brain a heaviness, the inert body weight of some curled and sleeping animal; but when she touched her head and pressed, the presence disappeared from the coordinates of actual space. Now it was in the top right corner of her mind, and in her imagination she could stand on tiptoe and raise her right hand to it.

It was important, however, not to provoke it; once this lazy creature moved from the peripheries to the center, then the knifing pains would obliterate all thought, and there would be no chance of dining with Leon and the family tonight. It bore her no malice, this animal, it was indifferent to her misery. It would move as a caged panther might: because it was awake, out of boredom, for the sake of movement itself, for no other reason at all, and with no awareness. She lay supine on her bed without a pillow, a glass of water within easy reach and, at her side, a book she knew she could not read. A long, blurred strip of daylight reflected on the ceiling above the pelmet was all that broke the darkness. She lay rigidly apprehensive, held at knifepoint, knowing that fear would not let her sleep and that her only hope was in keeping still.

The indistinct murmur of voices heard through a carpeted floor surpassed in clarity a typed-up transcript; a conversation that penetrated a wall or, better, two walls, came stripped of all but its essential twists and nuances. What to others would have been a muffling was to her alert senses, which were fine-tuned like the cat's whiskers of an old wireless, an almost unbearable amplification. She lay in the dark and knew everything. The less she was able to do, the more she was aware. But though she sometimes longed to rise up and intervene, especially if she thought Briony was in need of her, the fear of pain kept her in place. At worst, unrestrained, a matching set of sharpened kitchen knives would be drawn across her optic nerve, and then again, with greater downward pressure, and she would be entirely shut in and alone. Even groaning increased the agony. And so she lay there as the late afternoon slipped by".

My book also includes quotations from two classic texts. The first is *On Megrim, Sick Headache, and Some Allied Disorders* published in 1873 by Edward Liveing. His observations are remarkably accurate and remain relevant to this day.

Liveing describes many typical triggers, among them "...excessive brain-work, with a deficiency of bodily exercise, short restless nights, and insufficient sleep. By excessive brain-work I do not mean exclusively work of an intellectual kind, as in the close application of the mind to study literary composition, to the business of chambers or counting-house, but also that strain of the affective or emotional part of our nature, which is the result of prolonged mental anxiety, vexation, and disappointment, whether associated with the former or occurring independently and which is far more rapidly exhaustive of nervous power than any intellectual efforts which are free from such emotional complications."

A hundred years later, another great doctor, talented writer, and remarkable human being, Oliver Sacks, produced an extraordinary book on migraines, titled, simply, *Migraine.* It was first published in 1970 and remains in print. If you have an unusual or strange symptom that may be related to migraines, you will find it described in Sacks' book.

Do you really have migraines?

The official scientific definition of migraine is useful for research but in practice, it is a straitjacket. Many people do not fit this definition but they still have a migraine. According to the <u>third edition of The International Classification of Headache Disorders,</u> you have a migraine if you have at least two of the four features:

—unilateral pain

—moderate to severe intensity of pain

—worsening of pain with movement

—throbbing or pulsatile quality of pain.

Besides that, you have to have either:

—nausea with or without vomiting or

—sensitivity to light and noise.

The attack must last between 4 and 72 hours and you cannot have a brain tumor or another underlying medical condition (infectious, inflammatory, or hormonal disorder), causing these headaches.

In the real world, some people have throbbing pain with nausea, but no other features. Others have a mild headache with severe nausea and nothing else. Another common symptom of migraines not included in the official definition is the inability to function normally. The bottom line is that if you have any of the migraine features listed above, you have a migraine.

If you have a visual aura, you have a migraine regardless of the features of the headache that follows it. Auras occur in about 20% of people with migraine. It consists of partial loss of vision, flickering, or visual distortion. My aura is typical. I begin to see in the far periphery of my vision some wavy and flickering lines. Over the next 30 minutes, they slowly grow and occupy almost half of the visual field of each eye. I see them in the same half in each eye. This is why you may feel that the aura is in your left or right eye. Try to close one eye and you will realize that the same light show is happening in both eyes. Actually, the aura has little to do with your eyes. It is happening on one side of your brain. The first time you have an aura, many people think that they have a brain tumor. Fortunately, tumors are rare.

Sensory aura is less common. It is described as numbness or tingling that occurs on one side of the body. The numbness often begins in the hand, then skips to the face. At times, the entire half of the body goes numb. People with sensory aura often say that their arm or leg feels weak. On further questioning, it often turns out that the arm just feels awkward rather than weak. In some, the weakness of one side of the body does occur. We call this condition hemiplegic migraine. Aura of any kind lasts 10 to 60 minutes and most of the time precedes the onset of head pain. An aura can also occur in isolation, without a headache.

Neurologists divide migraines into episodic and chronic migraines. A person is considered to have a chronic migraine if she has at least 15 headache days a month and on eight of those days has migraine symptoms listed above. This is an arbitrary distinction and many people cycle from episodic into chronic and back into episodic phase.

After the collection of disability data on Danish and Russian patients, a new definition of chronic migraine has been proposed. It considers anyone having 8 or more migraine days each month to have chronic migraines. This may be important for research but not relevant for the treatment of individuals.

What I consider most relevant in practice is the degree of migraine-related disability. The frequency and other features are not as important. The more disabling the migraine, the more aggressive the treatment I undertake.

Many people ask me, what is the cause of migraines? We have evidence that genetic predisposition can play a role. This does not mean that if you have a certain genetic makeup, you are destined to suffer. Even if everyone in your family has migraines, you may find a way to control this disease. Genes make you more predisposed to migraines, but unlike some other genetic diseases, they do not guarantee that you will have attacks of migraine.

Migraine is often misdiagnosed. At the end of this book, I describe conditions that are often mistaken for migraine. The most common mistake is calling migraine a sinus or a tension-type headache. If you have a sinus headache, you will almost always have a colored nasal discharge. A small amount of clear discharge can happen with migraines. A tension-type headache will rarely bother you enough to make you read this book.

Look for triggers

Almost anyone can have a migraine given enough triggers. Combine lack of sleep, stress, dehydration, and alcohol, and 90% of people will develop a migraine. If you have a genetic predisposition, you may need only one or a few triggers. While avoiding triggers makes obvious sense, excessive fear of being exposed to them can lead to persistent anxiety and a self-fulfilling prophecy. This becomes much less of an issue if you can find a consistently effective acute treatment with a prescription drug or without. In some people, there are no easily identifiable triggers and migraines just happen for no obvious reason.

According to the company 23andme which collects genetic and other data from millions of people, these are the most common migraine triggers (most people have more than one trigger, so the percentages add up to much more than 100%):

—stress (85%)

—insufficient sleep (72%)

—dehydration (64%)

—looking at bright sunlight (61%)

—inhaling smoke/strong odors (57%)

—staring at a computer screen (56%)

—flashing or flickering lights (56%)

—weather changes (50%)

—low blood sugar (49%)

—loud environments (48%)

—heat (47%)

—caffeine withdrawal (43%)

—alcoholic beverages (42%)

—large groups of people (28%)

—bananas (6%)

They also listed treatments rated as most effective by patients with migraine

1. Dark, quiet room

2. Sleep

3. Eliminate red wine

4. Passage of time

5. Eliminate MSG

6. Avoid smoke

7. Wear sunglasses

Collecting massive amounts of data allowed 23andme to identify certain genes that predispose people to migraines. At this point, knowing which gene makes one predisposed is of no practical significance. We are far from being able to manipulate genes or even predict which treatment is likely to help and which one is likely to cause side effects. Such predictions based on genetic makeup are already being used in psychiatry and we hope that this will soon come to the field of migraines.

Keeping a diary, or not

Many headache specialists insist on patients keeping a headache diary. They consider it a part of a successful approach to managing migraine headaches. The diary can help identify potential migraine triggers and contributing factors while a description of specific symptoms can help tailor individual therapy. Most of my patients have been resistant to keeping a diary. They may have a good reason to resist.

A 2019 article published in *Wired* magazine *Why tracking your symptoms can make you feel worse,* cites research that suggests that keeping a diary of symptoms can indeed make one feel worse. This seems to be true across different conditions – insomnia, back pain, and also migraine. One possible explanation is that constantly paying attention to sensations in the body can magnify them. These sensations may send an alarm to the brain, oh-oh, a migraine is starting. This in turn leads to anxiety, activation of the fight-or-flight response, and soon a real migraine begins. Sometimes a patient comes in with pages and pages of diaries and notes that describe each migraine attack in great detail with every possible trigger, medications tried, and their side effects. I know that this patient will be harder to help because they are so deeply focused on their symptoms.

For migraine headaches, we have a good substitute for a daily diary. It is a Migraine Disability Assessment Scale, or MIDAS, which assesses migraine-related disability over the previous three months. This is a simple 5-question scale. It was validated by comparing a daily diary with patient recollection. Surprisingly, the correlation was strong and the scale gives reliable information. We ask patients to complete MIDAS on every visit. At a glance, it tells us how disabling the migraines are and how aggressive we need to be in starting preventive therapies, such as Botox, drugs, and the new monoclonal antibodies. This score is also helpful for patients who may not remember how disabling the headaches were before they started a particular treatment.

As far as identifying triggers, most are obvious and patients do not need a diary to tell them that triggers such as alcohol, lack of sleep, skipping meals, stress, are causing their attacks. I do not discourage anyone from keeping a diary. Some triggers are not obvious and a diary can help identify them. These include gluten sensitivity, weather factors, the menstrual cycle, and others. You may want to keep a diary for a few months and see if you can get any useful information from it.

When do you need testing?

You don't need an MRI or a CAT scan if your headaches have not changed for years or if several members of your family have similar headaches. A scan may be indicated if one or more of these are present:

—headaches are of recent onset

—the headaches are more severe than in the past

—fever

—pronounced neck stiffness

—weakness or numbness of one side of the face or body

—difficulty speaking

—visual problems

—fatigue

—dizziness

—confusion

—loss of consciousness

—muscle twitching

In the US, we do too many tests. Misapplied financial incentives and the threat of malpractice lawsuits are to blame. Tests and procedures are reimbursed at a much higher rate than the time spent talking to a patient. Although a detailed history and examination usually suffice, doctors are rushed and often order tests such as an MRI scan to reassure the patient and protect herself or himself against a lawsuit. Sometimes getting an MRI can be cost-effective and even therapeutic. Patients stop worrying about having a brain tumor and their migraines improve. They may also stop going to doctors. Although some ask for an MRI every year or two just to make sure.

Blood tests are much more useful than brain scans. I see many patients who had an MRI scan but not blood tests. Blood tests can detect problems that may persist undetected for years. These include deficiencies of magnesium, CoQ_{10}, vitamins B_{12} and D, thyroid dysfunction, anemia, celiac disease, abnormal glucose metabolism.

NON-DRUG APPROACHES

Environment

1. Air Pollution

An increase in air pollution correlates with an increase in visits to Canadian emergency rooms. The pollutants that showed this correlation include nitrogen dioxide, sulfur dioxide, and particles smaller than 2.5 μm. A similar study in Taiwan discovered that in addition to these three pollutants, ozone and carbon monoxide also correlated with clinic visits. Pollution also seems to contribute to the development of Alzheimer's and other dementias.

Besides moving to a place with a cleaner environment, you can buy an air purifier with a HEPA filter. If possible, avoid going outside when pollution is high. Daily air pollution levels are posted at World's Air Pollution: Real-time Air Quality Index. In the US you can also check it at http://www.airnow.gov.

2. Weather

Weather is a common trigger of migraine headaches. There are several possible weather-related triggers. They are high humidity, high temperature, drop in barometric pressure, and Chinook winds. Other types of strong local winds can bother some people with migraines as well. Mistral, Sirocco, Foehn, Haboob, Hamsin, Levant, Leveche are poetic-sounding names but these winds can bring misery to those with migraines.

Some migraine sufferers, just like many people with arthritis, can predict rainy weather. We suspect that a drop in barometric pressure could lead to a widening of blood vessels inside the skull and this may be a migraine trigger. Faulty regulation of blood vessel size in migraine patients could explain the sensitivity to barometric pressure changes. This problem with blood vessels may also explain exercise or sex-induced headaches. Whenever the blood vessels dilate excessively they trigger a migraine. High altitude headache or mountain sickness is another example of headaches caused by low barometric pressure. People living at high altitudes (like Denver) are more likely to have migraines than those living at sea level. Treatment of barometric pressure headaches begins with general health measures. A drug used for mountain sickness, acetazolamide can also prevent weather-related headaches. Take it when the barometric pressure drops. Such a drop precedes migraines by many hours. Some people can prevent a weather-related headache by taking ibuprofen or sumatriptan. Several apps can send you an alert when barometric pressure falls. This gives you time to take a preventive drug.

Acetazolamide can be also effective for people who develop migraines while flying. These headaches are often similar to weather-related headaches. Both may be caused by a drop in barometric pressure at high altitudes.

It is unclear how high humidity would cause a headache, but it often does.

High temperature may lead to a) dehydration, which is a trigger of migraines for many and b) again, dilatation of blood vessels which the body uses to cool itself by bringing more warm blood to the surface (this is why we look red in the heat).

3. Light

Bright light is a common trigger of migraine headaches. Some people report having their migraines triggered by a single flash of the sun reflecting on water or window glass. Besides wearing dark sunglasses, there are general measures that lower your brain's excitability, including sleep, exercise, meditation, and most of the measures mentioned in this book.

Fluorescent lights produce an imperceptible flicker that can trigger a migraine. Use incandescent lights where possible. If you work in a shared space, see if the fluorescent bulb above your desk can be taken out. Replace it with a desk lamp. FL-41 filters (see below) reduce the intensity of the flicker. Halogen lights do not flicker, but their brightness can be a problem as well.

Low-blue-light glasses

Many migraine sufferers get an attack when they spend time outdoors. Sometimes an overcast sky is worse than a cloudless one. Orange-colored lenses block the blue part of the spectrum. They can reduce the risk of migraine caused by daylight. Others find orange lenses irritating. Try them on in an eyeglass store. If they feel soothing, they are likely to help.

FL-41 tint

Rose-tinted "FL-41" lenses reduce the frequency of migraine attacks by filtering out the part of the light spectrum that some migraine patients are sensitive to. In a study of 20 children, half were given rose-tinted (FL-41) glasses and the other half, blue-tinted ones. They were told to wear them mostly in school where fluorescent lights are widely used. After four months, the attack frequency in the rose tint group dropped from 6.2 to 1.6. There was no improvement in the blue tint group. Four of the 10 children in the blue tint group dropped out of the study early. This tint can be applied by an optician to any prescription lens. Non-prescription glasses with an FL-41 tint are also available from several manufacturers.

Green ambient light

According to a study published in *Brain*, by a leading headache researcher, Dr. Rami Burstein, all colors of the spectrum worsen pain perception, except for green. Blue light produces the strongest pain response. This explains why wearing orange-colored lenses that block the blue light can help some people. Another paper by Burstein and his colleagues at Harvard published in the *Proceedings of the National Academy of Sciences* suggests that exposure to green light also has a positive effect on mood and other brain functions. Dr. Burstein developed the Allay lamp that emits a pure green light (about 530 nm). My patients find it calming and pain-relieving. A regular bulb painted green will not do. It lets out colors other than pure green.

4. Noise

Sensitivity to noise is one of the defining features of migraine headaches. If you live in a noisy neighborhood you may consider installing sound-proof windows. Wearing noise-canceling earphones is another option. Listening to pleasant music or white noise can help. Fortunately, noise-canceling earphones have become inexpensive. You can also buy inexpensive ear muffs made by gun manufacturers. However, sometimes prolonged pressure from earphones can also trigger an attack. If you are invited to a party with loud music, remember to bring earplugs.

5. Odors

Noxious smells such as car exhaust, gasoline, paint, cleaning chemicals, and smoke are a powerful trigger for some people. Certain types of perfume and the scent of flowers can also bring on a migraine. Besides avoiding such smells and improving your general health, carry a vial of peppermint or lavender oil. Smell it to block a bad odor. Have the courage to ask your friends and family not to wear perfume when you are spending time with them.

6. Mold and allergies

We are constantly exposed to molds indoors and outdoors. But only exposure to high levels of certain types of molds can make you sick. An allergic reaction to mold can cause a runny nose, sneezing, nasal congestion, watery eyes, skin rash, itching, and difficulty breathing. Headaches are also common. Chronic rhinitis or inflammation and swelling of the mucous membrane of the nose are characterized by a runny nose and stuffiness. It can be the result of allergies and is associated with an increase in the frequency and disability of migraine headaches.

Food

In the book mentioned above, Edward Liveing advises migraine sufferers to "eat little" and suggests "exchanging a highly nutritious regimen for a much lighter dietary".

As mentioned above, dehydration is the third common migraine trigger. Some people have a faulty thirst mechanism. They can go all day without drinking fluids and not feeling thirsty. These people need to constantly remind themselves to drink. And if they do, their migraines improve. I call it a water cure.

7. Sugar

Sugar is not always an obvious trigger. Many people develop a migraine hours after a carbohydrate-rich food. Three-quarters of people with migraine have reactive hypoglycemia. This means that their blood sugar drops too low after eating a carbohydrate-rich meal.

People with migraines also have a higher incidence of insulin resistance. This means that your cells need more than normal amounts of insulin to utilize sugar in your blood. Signs of insulin resistance include obesity, elevated triglyceride levels in the blood, high fasting blood sugar levels, high blood pressure, and others.

We have evidence that a ketogenic diet may help improve migraines. A few of my patients who have tried it, also found it effective. The ketogenic diet is hard to adhere to for more than a month or two. It is more realistic to try a low-carb diet that is not as stringent regarding eating carbs. It is not only desserts but sweet fruit and fruit juices that contain large amounts of sugar. You can safely eat all kinds of berries, sour cherries, and green apples.

8. Salt

Eating more salt leads to more headaches, according to a study published in *BMJ Open*. In a multicenter feeding study with three 30-day periods, 390 participants were randomized to two different diets. One was the DASH diet (Dietary Approaches to Stop Hypertension, a diet rich in fruits, vegetables, and low-fat dairy products with reduced saturated and total fat). The second diet was regular and not healthy. On their assigned diet (DASH or regular), participants ate food with high sodium during one period, intermediate sodium during another period, and low sodium during another period, in random order. The occurrence of headaches was similar on DASH and the control diet. However, when either diet contained less sodium, headaches were fewer. There was no correlation between elevated blood pressure and headaches.

A study published in the journal Headache by researchers at Stanford and UCLA specifically looked at the possible connection between salt intake and migraines. This was a national nutritional study that examined sodium intake in people with a history of migraine or severe headaches. The study included 8,819 adults with reliable data on diet and headache history. Dietary sodium intake was measured using reliable estimates.

Unlike the *BMJ Open* study, this one found that higher dietary intake of sodium was associated with a lower chance of migraines or severe headaches. This relationship was not affected by age or sex. In women, this inverse relationship was limited to those with lower weight (as measured by body mass index, or BMI), while in men the relationship did not differ by BMI.

Considering that eating more salt is safe for healthy people, you may want to temporarily increase your salt intake. I would suggest adding table salt to a healthy and balanced diet, rather than eating salty foods such as smoked fish, potato chips, processed deli meats, or pickles. These foods contain sulfites, nitrites, and other preservatives which can trigger a migraine attack.

Do not increase your salt intake if you have high blood pressure and kidney or heart disease.

9. Gluten

Celiac disease is more common in migraine patients. The reverse is also true. Migraines are much more common in those with celiac disease. Researchers at Columbia University showed that chronic headaches were present in 30% of those with celiac disease, 56% with gluten sensitivity, 23% with inflammatory bowel disease, and 14% of control subjects. Celiac disease is a severe autoimmune disease caused by a wheat allergy. It affects about 3 million Americans. The estimates of gluten sensitivity run as high as 18 million. Many doctors are skeptical about the existence of non-celiac gluten sensitivity. The evidence indicates that this is a real condition. Gluten sensitivity is mediated through a different type of allergy than in celiac disease. There is nothing to lose by trying a gluten-free diet. Strictly adhere to it for several weeks to see if your migraines improve. People often report that stopping gluten gives them more energy and makes them feel better overall.

10. Dairy

Lactose intolerance can cause headaches. However, headaches are rarely the main symptom. Most people figure out that they are lactose intolerant because they also have bloating, gas, stomach pains, and diarrhea.

Aged cheese has been reported to be a migraine trigger by 18% of 490 patients. These people may not have lactose intolerance. They react to the fermentation products in cheese. Yogurt is also fermented and can be a trigger. Cottage cheese is safe.

11. Food allergies

Many people suspect that food allergies cause headaches. When certain foods cause a migraine, it is usually not due to an allergic reaction, but due to a chemical reaction. An allergy occurs when the body's immune defense mechanisms try to isolate and attack an offending substance. This substance is called an allergen. It is possible to evaluate this immune response by measuring blood levels of immune globulins (IgG) specific to a particular food or substance. Because there are so many different foods, hundreds of tests are required. Doing such extensive and expensive testing has been controversial. People with irritable bowel syndrome who had high levels of IgG to certain foods improved after eliminating those foods. Another way to detect food allergies is by a scratch test. This is done by placing an extract of different foods into skin scratches. The skin reaction is then measured.

A sophisticated study published in Cephalalgia by Dr. Ertas and his colleagues looked at food allergies in migraine patients. They tested IgG levels to 266 foods in the blood of 30 migraine sufferers. The number of foods these 30 patients were allergic to ranged from 13 to 35. After testing, each patient ate a diet that included or excluded foods they were allergic to for six weeks. After that, they had two weeks of an unrestricted diet. This was followed by another 6 weeks of the opposite diet – if they first had a diet free of allergen, then they were switched to a diet with allergens and vice versa. Neither the doctor nor the patient knew what foods the patient was allergic to or which diet was given in each 6-week period. The study showed that significantly fewer migraines occurred when the diet excluded foods patients were allergic to. This is the first rigorous study to suggest that food allergy testing may be of use.

12. Tyramine

Aged cheeses contain more tyramine than cream cheese and tyramine is what had been suspected to be the trigger of migraines. Other foods with large amounts of tyramine include fermented sausages, sliced meat products, chicken liver, beer, red wine, and some fruits, such as raspberries and bananas. In one study, eating pure tyramine by migraine patients did not trigger any attacks. The authors allowed for the possibility that tyramine may be a contributing factor but not the sole trigger. This is true with most triggers. The more of them you pile on, the more likely you will develop a migraine attack.

13. Monosodium glutamate, nitrates, nitrites, sulfites

Monosodium glutamate (MSG) is a flavor enhancer. I tell my patients only half-jokingly that if something tastes very good, it must have MSG in it. In a study of 9,427 female migraineurs, 25% listed MSG as either a trigger or factor that worsened their migraine. A study investigating the effect of MSG consumption in 14 healthy subjects showed that 8 out of 14 developed a headache from MSG. Only 2 out of 14 developed it from placebo.

Unfortunately, MSG is often disguised under a large number of names: vegetable protein, textured protein, soy protein, yeast extract, glutamic acid, monopotassium glutamate, calcium glutamate, monoammonium glutamate, magnesium glutamate calcium caseinate, and others.

We have no studies of the effect of foods containing nitrates, nitrites, and sulfites. These substances are also suspected to trigger migraine attacks. They are present in dried, pickled, smoked, fermented, cured, and processed foods. It is a good idea to try to avoid eating them for a few weeks to see if migraines improve.

14. Caffeine

Caffeine helps relieve migraine headaches but it can also worsen them. A double-blind study published in the *New England Journal of Medicine* proved that caffeine withdrawal causes headaches. This is no surprise to anyone who cannot get their usual *venti* or *trenta* cup from Starbucks. We do know that caffeine withdrawal causes headaches. Some patients tell me that they get a headache when they drink coffee. A study published by Harvard researchers in *The American Journal of Medicine* addressed this unexamined question – does drinking coffee directly trigger a migraine?

This was a high-quality study. It showed a significant association between the number of caffeinated beverages and the odds of developing a migraine on that day. This association was stronger in people who normally drank 1-2 cups of coffee daily. They were more likely to get a migraine on days when they drank 3 or more cups. Even after accounting for daily alcohol intake, stress, sleep, activity, and menstrual bleeding, 1-2 servings of caffeinated beverages were not associated with an increased risk of developing a headache. Three or more servings were. The researchers also considered the possibility of reverse causation, meaning that people might have drank coffee to treat a headache. This was not the case.

My advice is to drink not more than 1 or 2 small cups of coffee a day. During a migraine attack having an extra cup along with your usual medication may provide additional relief. The beneficial effects of caffeine on migraines is described in the drug section of this book.

15. Alcohol

Alcohol gives you a flush and makes you feel warm because it opens blood vessels. This is one reason why alcohol can trigger a migraine. The other is chemicals in alcohol such as sulfites, tyramine, and fermentation products. Vodka, tequila, and white wine have less of these chemicals and are less likely to cause headaches. You may want to avoid red wine, scotch, bourbon, champagne, and beer.

But this is not so straightforward. The French argue that it is white and not red wine that is more likely to cause a migraine.

Resveratrol, an ingredient in red wine may be responsible for the health benefits of red wine. The researchers have found that resveratrol has the potential to relieve pain. When I blogged about one such study, I received many interesting comments. Some people reported that taking resveratrol caused a migraine. But here are a few of the positive comments about drinking wine that you can still find on my blog. "I had a massive headache and drunk a glass of red wine and the headache is gone WOW", "3 sips of wine takes away my barometric pressure migraine and I feel so happy", "I find that red wine reduces my migraine headache. It's nice to know I'm not alone on this", "After a migraine building all day, I had a glass of red wine, which lately has been my only relief from migraines".

16. Fasting and weight loss (5)

Scientific studies show a direct correlation between the frequency and severity of headaches and the weight of a patient. One possible explanation is that an excess of fatty tissue promotes inflammation. The effect of weight loss on migraine is similar when it is achieved with bariatric surgery or behavioral intervention. The relief of migraines with weight loss occurs in adults and children.

Many migraine patients report getting a headache if they don't eat on time. People who don't have migraines can develop a tension-type headache from not eating. One study showed that nighttime snacking reduces the chance of a migraine attack.

A drop in glucose level during intense mental activity could explain migraines under stress. The brain mass is only 5% of the body's weight but it consumes 20% of the body's energy.

Fasting for one to several days has many health benefits but it can be a migraine trigger. Intermittent fasting is much easier to do and has similar benefits according to a review in *The New England Journal of Medicine*. It consists of eating all your meals within a 6-8 hour window. Have your breakfast at 10, lunch at 2, and dinner at 6. Intermittent fasting is less likely to trigger a migraine. Unless you need a nighttime snack to prevent an attack.

Exercise

17. Aerobic, high-intensity interval training, strength-building (8)

Strong scientific evidence indicates that aerobic (cardio) exercise improves migraines and other headaches. A Swedish study of 91 patients established that exercising for 40 minutes 3 times a week is as effective as relaxation training or taking a preventive migraine drug topiramate. Topiramate, however, caused significant side effects.

Another study by the same group of 46,648 people found a strong inverse correlation between physical activity and the frequency of headaches.

High-intensity interval training (HIT) has been gaining in popularity since the 1980s because it provides all of the benefits of exercise in a shorter time.

A study by Swiss researchers compared the effect of HIT with moderate-intensity continuous training (MCT) and with no exercise at all on the number of migraine headache days. Patients in the HIT group did 4 periods of intensive exercise (90% of maximum intensity) each lasting 4 minutes, separated by 3 minutes of exercise at 70% of maximum. The moderate-intensity exercise was done at 70% for 45 minutes. Both groups exercised twice a week. Both types of exercise reduced the number of migraine headache days, but HIT was more effective. HIT also improved the condition of blood vessels. The MCT did not.

Strength training may be as good as aerobic exercise. Just like intense aerobic exercise, it boosts the release of brain-derived neurotrophic factor (BDNF), a neurotransmitter that is crucial for the normal functioning of brain cells. The release of BDNF during intense exercise could be responsible for many benefits of exercise, including the prevention of migraines. A study by Danish researchers of 573 office workers showed that one weekly hour of high-intensity strength training reduces headache frequency and severity.

18. Neck exercise (4)

Many people have neck pain with their migraines. Some patients tell me that neck pain precedes an attack of migraine. Sometimes pain begins in the upper back, travels to the neck, and then blooms into a severe migraine. Migraine can also cause neck pain. This can lead to a vicious cycle of neck pain contributing to the headache and headache worsening the neck pain. Sitting in front of a computer or staring at a cellphone for hours can strain the neck and contribute to migraine headaches. Proper posture and upper back and neck exercises help.

Try to remember doing a chin tuck all day long. Isometric neck exercises take a minute to do and if repeated throughout the day, can prevent headaches. Here is how you do it. Using the palm of your hand apply pressure for 10 seconds to the front, back, and sides of the head while resisting this pressure with your neck muscles. This takes only 40 seconds. Try to do it frequently throughout the day. You may want to add a few slow deep breaths to lower tension in your entire body.

19. The Feldenkrais method (3)

Moshe Feldenkrais, a physicist who was living and working in Paris in the 1930s injured his knee. The surgeon he consulted gave him a 50% chance of success from an operation. These odds did not appeal to Feldenkrais. He decided to investigate the body mechanics and figured out a way to heal his knee. This was the start of what became the Feldenkrais method. After a few years, Feldenkrais quit his successful engineering career to devote the rest of his life to teaching his method around the world. His method is still being used, though not as widely as it deserves to be. The idea is to retrain the control of muscles by the brain rather than by trying to work on muscles directly. The method is gentle, deceptively simple, and can be dramatically effective.

Feldenkrais did not call it therapy and always insisted that he did not treat patients, but taught lessons on how to move naturally. His lessons often led to a dramatic relief of pain, improved movement, and better functioning. This method can help symptoms of cerebral palsy, stroke, multiple sclerosis, back, and neck pain. Feldenkrais felt that the key to healing was to become aware of what one is doing. Dancers, artists, and athletes have been using Feldenkrais lessons to improve their performance and to avoid and heal injuries. In the early 1950s, Feldenkrais worked with the first Prime Minister of Israel, David Ben-Gurion. Ben-Gurion's decades-long chronic back pain dramatically improved. Feldenkrais quit his position as the first director of the electronics department of the Israeli Defense Force and decided to devote all of his time to teaching his movement method. He trained hundreds of practitioners around the world and they in turn trained the next generation of teachers.

Jane Brody, a long-time health columnist for the *New York Times* described her positive experience in *Trying the Feldenkrais Method for Chronic Pain*.

The Feldenkrais method emphasizes gentle and often small movements that re-educate and re-establish the connection between the body and the brain. It also makes you do movements that do not come naturally and that we never do, such as turning your head to one side and moving your eyes in the opposite direction. It is difficult to describe this method in words, but even a single lesson can show its healing potential.

Try this simple exercise. Check the range of movements in your neck – how far can you turn your head to one side, then the other without straining. Then, put palms of your hands on your cheeks and press your arms to your body. Now, turn your body at the waist from the midline to the left and return back to the midline. Go only as far as it is comfortable to do. Repeat this 10 times. Then turn from the midline to the right and back 10 times. Now, put down your arms and test your range of movements again. Most people will notice a significant improvement. This is surprising because it happens without moving the neck. You can <u>watch me doing this</u> exercise on YouTube. I also show <u>another exercise</u> that improves the lateral flexion of your neck.

Here is a possible explanation of how Feldenkrais works. The visual cues have a much stronger impact on the brain than from proprioception. Proprioception is the information sent to the brain from our muscles, ligaments, and joints. <u>When vision and proprioception are incongruent, the brain relies first on vision and then proprioception</u>. When your eyes indicate that your head moved far to one side, the brain cannot tell if the movement came from turning the torso or the neck. Repeating the move from the torso trains your brain to expect your head and eyes to go so far. The next time, when you move your neck and not the torso, the brain lets the neck muscles go farther.

And there is another fascinating phenomenon that supports this explanation. When we cross our hands, we feel less pain in the hand. *The Journal of Pain* published the article <u>"Seeing One's Own Painful Hand Positioned in the Contralateral Space Reduces Subjective Reports of Pain..."</u>. The results of functional MRI imaging of the brain looking at this phenomenon was reported in another article in the same journal: <u>Crossing the line of pain: FMRI correlates of crossed-hands analgesia.</u> Our visual cues are important to our ability to move and feel pain and this may be one of the ways the Feldenkrais method improves movement and relieves pain.

If individual Feldenkrais lessons are too expensive, try group lessons. You can also learn it by reading books and watching YouTube videos. I recorded and posted on YouTube some neck exercises that improve the range of neck movements. Besides the exercises to improve <u>side-to-side</u> and <u>lateral movements</u>, I also recorded an effective <u>exercise to relieve upper back tension</u>.

20. Yoga (4)

I love hot yoga, but the intense heat is not for everyone. If you've ever done yoga you will not need convincing that it may very well help prevent migraine headaches. A <u>study published by Indian doctors in 2020 in the leading neurological journal, *Neurology*</u> examined the effect of yoga as add-on therapy to the conventional medical treatment of migraine headaches. It was a "prospective, randomized, open-label superiority trial with blinded endpoint assessment carried out at a single tertiary care academic hospital in New Delhi". One hundred and sixty patients with episodic migraine were randomly assigned to medical and yoga groups. A total of 114 patients completed the trial. Compared to medical therapy, the yoga group showed a significant reduction in: 1) headache frequency; 2) headache intensity; 3) disability as measured by the headache impact test (HIT-6); 4) migraine disability assessment (MIDAS) score; and 5) in the number of pills taken.

The authors concluded that: "Yoga as add-on therapy in migraine is superior to medical therapy alone. It may be useful to integrate a cost-effective and safe intervention like yoga into the management of migraine."

A word of caution: Migraine sufferers are more prone to a dissection of arteries in the neck. This condition is described at the end of this book. Try to avoid extreme twisting or bending of your neck, doing headstands or shoulder stands. Forcing your neck into extreme positions can also cause herniation of a disc in your spine. I've found standing on my head strangely pleasant. But this can be dangerous. The bones in the cervical spine are relatively small and fragile. They were not intended to carry the weight of our bodies. On the other hand, a proper headstand should not involve any pressure on your head – all of the weight is supposed to rest on the forearms. Some people prone to migraines cannot tolerate any inversion poses where the head is lower than the heart.

21. Eye movement exercises (3)

Many brain disorders can impair the control of eye movements. This can lead to incorrect information being passed from the eyes to the brain. This in turn can worsen brain dysfunction. Eye strain can also contribute to migraines and post-concussion headaches.

A <u>study by New Zealand doctors published in the journal</u> *Brain* <u>showed</u> <u>that 3 to 5 months after a concussion, eye movement difficulties</u> were still present. These difficulties were not affected by the presence of depression or degree of intellectual ability. Compared with neuropsychological tests, eye movements were more likely to be markedly impaired in patients with many post-concussion symptoms.

To diagnose eye movement problems, infrared eye-tracking equipment is often used. One of the companies offering such equipment is RightEye. Their computer tests various types of eye movements (smooth pursuit, vertical and horizontal saccades), gaze fixation, reading, reaction time, and other functions.

<u>The symptoms of concussion</u> improve with eye movement exercises. A review of several published studies of vision therapy for post-concussion symptoms found it "promising."

Physical methods

22. Acupuncture (5)

Acupuncture has been tested in a large number of clinical trials. Dr. Zhang, a neurologist at Stanford and two of his colleagues <u>published a review of trials</u> <u>that compared acupuncture with standard pharmacological migraine therapy</u>. This review included only rigorous trials that compared the efficacy of acupuncture with a standard migraine preventive medication in patients with chronic or episodic migraines.

Out of the 706 published reports, seven clinical trials with a total of 1430 participants were of high quality. The types of acupuncture and pharmacological treatments varied from trial to trial. This made it difficult to make any sweeping conclusions. However, several of the studies revealed acupuncture to be more effective than the standard pharmacological treatments.

One of the leading German neurologists, <u>Christoph Diener in an editorial</u> <u>in the journal of the International Headache Society,</u> *Cephalalgia* <u>wrote</u> that "Despite this poor evidence, acupuncture was the most frequently used method to treat primary headaches in many European countries." In the same editorial, he reviewed two very large government-funded trials of acupuncture. He wrote, "...acupuncture is as effective as drug therapy, but ...sham acupuncture is as effective as 'real' acupuncture." And, "...acupuncture should be offered to patients who do not respond to prophylactic treatment with drugs, terminate drug treatment because of adverse events or have contraindications to drug treatment."

Even if acupuncture is only as effective as drugs, its safety makes it a superior choice. The major drawbacks of acupuncture are that it is time-consuming and relatively expensive when compared to generic prescription drugs. The effect of acupuncture does not last a long time. To maintain the effect you may need to continue having it done every week or two.

23. Reflexology and massage (4)

The healer must be acquainted with many things and assuredly with rubbing.

—Hippocrates

Reflexology is a fancy name for foot massage. Just like body massage, it works well for some people. If you enjoy getting a massage you will not need any double-blind studies to convince you of its benefit. Double-blind studies are impossible, but compared to a control group, <u>weekly massage prevents migraines and improves sleep</u>. A <u>comparison of reflexology with body massage</u> showed them to be equally effective at relieving migraines.

Thai, Swedish, deep-tissue, shiatsu, and craniosacral are some of the popular types of massage. The skill and the talent of the person performing the massage are more important than the type of massage they are performing.

24. Chiropractic (4)

Chiropractors can also relieve migraines if they are skilled and talented. Norwegian researchers conducted a study of chiropractic manipulation for migraine headaches in 104 patients. They divided patients into three groups. One group received real chiropractic manipulation of the spine, another one received a sham treatment that consisted of just putting pressure over the shoulders and lower back, and the third group continued their usual medication. The real and sham chiropractic groups received 12 treatment sessions over 12 weeks. Patients were followed for a year. After 12 weeks patients in all three study groups reported improvement. However, a year later, only the chiropractic groups still felt better. On average, they had about four migraine days a month, down from six to eight before the treatment started.

Patients who continued their medications lost all of their improvement and their migraine frequency was back where it was at the baseline.

The results published in the *European Journal of Neurology* suggest that chiropractic is indeed effective in reducing migraine frequency. However, it also suggests that any hands-on treatment is equally effective. This probably explains the popularity of chiropractic, physical therapy, massage, reflexology, Reiki, energy therapies, and other hands-on treatments.

The same word of caution applies to chiropractic as to yoga. Avoid high-velocity adjustment – sudden upward pulling and twisting of the head. It carries a small but not negligible risk of stroke due to a dissection of an artery which is described at the end of this book. I was once consulted on an older man in an emergency department who was found to have a subdural hematoma (bleeding inside the skull) after receiving a chiropractic neck adjustment.

25. Music (2)

Music relieves experimental pain in healthy volunteers who are paid to endure pain and music. In one study, 18 volunteers were subjected to pleasant music, unpleasant music, and a silent period. Heat-induced pain was reduced only by pleasant music.

Children with migraines exposed to music improved as much as those given butterbur extract. Both groups improved more than a control group.

Music relieved the pain of osteoarthritis in the elderly. Those who listened to music for 20 minutes a day felt better than those who sat quietly for 20 minutes.

A study of 20 volunteers showed that both happy and sad melodies reduced heat pain. Listening to a lecture did not.

Another group of researchers examined the potential pain-relieving properties of three aspects of music: arousal, valence, and depth. Arousing music is characterized as "intense, forceful, abrasive, or thrilling". Valence refers to "fun, happy, lively, enthusiastic, and joyful". Depth means "intelligent, sophisticated, inspiring, complex, poetic, deep, emotional, and thoughtful." The degree of arousal and the depth of music had a greater effect on pain than valence. The authors concluded, "With the advent of online music streaming services, this research opens new possibilities for music-based pain interventions."

When I blogged about the effect of music on pain, I assumed that one of the comments was by a young man. He reported that hard rock music relieved his migraines. This suggests that music with high arousal may be indeed effective. I suspect that most people prefer calmer music.

26. Virtual reality (2)

A group of Italian researchers tested the effects of visual distraction on pain. They compared a classical hospital waiting room with an ideal room with a sea view. Both were represented in virtual reality (VR). They measured pain and brain responses induced by painful laser stimuli in healthy volunteers and patients with chronic migraine. Pain was induced in the right hand of sixteen chronic migraine patients and 16 healthy controls. This was done during a fully immersive VR experience, where two types of waiting rooms were simulated. Patients with migraine showed a reduction of laser pain rating and brain responses during the sea view simulation. Control subjects experienced the same level of pain in both types of simulated rooms.

Another study of 30 patients with chronic pain showed that 20 patients had pain relief during the VR session. Ten of them reported complete pain relief. Of the 20 who had relief, ten had continued relief after the VR session.

A combination of VR with biofeedback provided lasting benefits in nine of the ten children with chronic headaches who completed 10 training sessions.

About 5% to 10% of people who try VR get cybersickness, which is a feeling of dizziness or vertigo, similar to motion sickness.

There are several possible approaches to the treatment of pain using VR. One is by using VR for distraction. Another, by utilizing VR to facilitate biofeedback, which is proven to relieve migraine and tension headaches. The third way, yet to be proven, is by altering body perception.

27. Tai Chi (3)

This ancient Chinese martial art and form of exercise has many health benefits. In a study of Tai Chi in women with episodic migraines, 40 of them performed these exercises. They were compared to 33 women in the control group. The exercises were performed for one hour, five days a week, for twelve weeks.

The study showed that Tai Chi resulted in a significant, 3.6 day reduction in migraine days compared to the control group. The Tai Chi group also had a reduction in their blood pressure.

28. Dental appliances (3)

Many people who have migraine headaches also have jaw pain or a temporomandibular joint disorder (TMJ or TMD). This often results from clenching or grinding teeth at night. Some people clench their teeth throughout the day as well. Mental tension often brings on both migraines and teeth clenching.

A custom-made oral appliance can prevent migraines, according to a report by Scottish dentists. Such an appliance also prevents grinding of the teeth but not necessarily clenching.

A unique type of appliance is placed only on the front teeth. It can prevent clenching as well as grinding. If used for a long time, however, it can negatively affect teeth alignment.

Biofeedback has been shown to relieve both migraines and TMJ. Other treatments that can help are anti-inflammatory drugs, antidepressants, and Botox injections.

In some people, arthritis of the TMJ may require surgical treatment.

29. Care of nasal sinuses (2)

Migraines are often mistaken for sinus headaches. However, they are easy to differentiate. If you have green or yellow discharge from your nose, you have a sinus infection and a sinus headache. If the discharge with a severe headache is clear, the headache is almost always a migraine. This is not to say that allergies with nasal congestion have nothing to do with migraines. An irritation of nasal passages can trigger a migraine. Taking care of your sinuses by treating allergies can prevent migraine attacks. If you are prone to sinus infections, irrigate your sinuses using a Neti pot or a spray bottle. Using a humidifier when the air is dry can also help your sinuses.

Sleep

Going to sleep at the same time and getting up at the same time, including on weekends, is helpful for many migraine sufferers. Some feel frustrated because they look forward to getting extra sleep over the weekend. Instead of getting extra rest, sleeping late gives them a migraine. You can try taking a nap in the afternoon but keep it under an hour.

The other two causes of the weekend attacks are a delay in the first dose of caffeine and letdown from the week's stress.

30. Sleep apnea

Sleep apnea means a disruption of oxygen delivery to the lungs. It can happen from a brain disorder when it is called central sleep apnea. More often it is due to the collapse of airways in sleep. This is called obstructive sleep apnea. Obstructive sleep apnea often occurs in overweight people. A bed partner can often report snoring and episodes of gasping for air in the middle of the night. Sleep apnea results in poor quality of sleep. People have difficulty waking up in the morning and feel tired all day.

An overnight stay in a sleep laboratory can confirm the diagnosis. In the past few years, take-home devices have become almost as accurate.

If you are overweight, treatment of sleep apnea begins with an attempt at weight loss.

Another approach is to use an oral appliance that moves the lower jaw forward. This prevents the tongue from falling back and obstructing the airway. An examination by an ear-nose-throat (ENT) specialist may reveal excessive tissue around the tonsils that may be obstructing the flow of air. Removing this extra tissue by surgery can help.

If none of these measures are applicable or don't help, a CPAP (continuous positive airway pressure) machine can make a big difference. Over the years these machines have become smaller, quieter, and more comfortable.

Many people cannot tolerate even the newer CPAP machines. Such people may benefit from <u>Inspire, an implantable upper airway stimulation device</u> that coordinates the opening and the closing of airways to improve the delivery of oxygen.

31. Restless leg syndrome

Restless leg syndrome (RLS) is a common condition that often goes undiagnosed. This is in part because RLS begins in childhood and often runs in the family. It is not perceived as an illness. Sometimes the diagnosis of RLS is easy to make. A person who constantly shakes his or her foot usually has it. In some people, excessive leg or body movements occur only in sleep. Then the diagnosis is less obvious. Speaking to the bed partner helps. They are the ones who are constantly kicked and woken up by these movements.

Iron and vitamin B_{12} deficiencies can cause RLS symptoms. These two deficiencies need to be ruled out first. A sleep study is done to confirm the diagnosis. This involves an overnight stay at a sleep laboratory. During the test, wires are attached to the scalp, monitors measure the breathing, and a video camera records movements of the legs and body.

By disrupting sleep, RLS may increase the frequency and severity of migraines.

A study of 505 headache patients by Taiwanese neurologists showed that with an increase in migraine frequency the occurrence of RLS is also increased. This connection is particularly pronounced in those who have migraines with auras. Anxiety and sleep disturbance were also associated with RLS.

Women with migraines are 20% more likely to have RLS, according to a study that involved 31,370 women. Fortunately, we have many effective drugs to treat RLS – ropinirole (Requip), pramipexole (Mirapex), gabapentin (Neurontin). If those drugs do not work, opioid drugs, such as hydrocodone or oxycodone can be extremely effective. These drugs are usually taken before going to sleep. This means that they are less likely to cause a high that can lead to addiction. The more common problem is the development of tolerance – needing to keep increasing the dose to achieve the same results. If tolerance becomes a problem, the drug should be slowly discontinued. We usually have patients sign an opioid agreement described in the section on preventive drugs.

32. Insomnia

Insomnia is more common in people with migraines than in those without. Depression and anxiety are more common in migraineurs. These conditions often lead to insomnia. Surveys indicate that 38% of migraine sufferers sleep less than 6 hours, compared to 10% of the general population.

Most people are reluctant to start taking sleep medications. They are understandably concerned about becoming dependent on medicine, being sleepy the next day, having other short-term and long-term side effects. Some of the preventive drugs listed in the second half of this book can improve sleep. These include some antidepressants and muscle relaxants.

Fortunately, non-drug therapies can be as effective. For many, natural remedies, such as magnesium, valerian root, and melatonin work well without causing any side effects.

A good approach to treating insomnia is cognitive-behavioral therapy (CBT). Psychologists at the University of Mississippi showed that behavioral treatments can be effective in relieving insomnia and improving chronic migraines. The researchers compared CBT specifically developed for insomnia with sham treatment. After two weeks of intervention, headaches improved in the sham group more than the active group, but six weeks later, headache frequency dropped by 49% in the active group and 25% in the sham group. Improvement in insomnia symptoms strongly correlated with headache frequency. The CBT group had a significant increase in total sleep time and the quality of sleep.

A large body of evidence indicates that behavioral therapies do relieve insomnia. It is no surprise that better sleep is associated with fewer headaches since sleep deprivation is a common migraine trigger. Cost and access to a CBT therapist can be a problem. Several online programs are inexpensive and effective. The coaching and human contact factor still make a live therapist preferable.

Another simple method I've used over the years whenever I cannot fall asleep is visualization or guided imagery. Instead of using only visual images, you need to engage all of your senses. For example, with your eyes closed, imagine yourself in a place where you tend to feel relaxed – lying on a beach, on a cool lawn, on a float in a pool, or in a green forest. Visualize all the details and also hear the sound of the breeze or waves, smell the fresh sea air or the grass, feel the touch of the wind or sand. At first, it takes effort. But if you keep going to the same place every time, after a while you will fall asleep within minutes. Here you can find more detailed instructions for this method.

Through the use of brain scans, scientists have been able to see that imagining a thing, a place, or a situation elicits the same changes in the brain as actually experiencing it. Whatever physiological changes are associated with the real experience may also occur just by imagining it. The more vividly you imagine the situation through visual images, odors, physical sensations, and sounds, the more powerful the physical response. This means that imagining a relaxing situation – a day at the beach, for example – can bring on the same physical reactions as actually experiencing that situation.

Supplements

Migraines can be caused by deficiencies in one or more vital nutrients. For this reason, vitamin and mineral supplements can help relieve migraines. There are many causes of these deficiencies. Many people eat an unhealthy diet that is low in vegetables and high in sugar. Poor absorption of nutrients due to gastrointestinal problems such as irritable bowel syndrome, celiac disease, and colitis is also a common cause of deficiencies that contribute to migraine. Long-term intake of acid-lowering medications can cause vitamin B_{12} and other deficiencies. These drugs include proton pump inhibitors (PPIs) such as omeprazole (Prilosec), pantoprazole (Protonix), and esomeprazole (Nexium) and H_2 blockers that include ranitidine (Zantac), famotidine (Pepcid) and cimetidine (Tagamet).

Acid-lowering drugs taken for longer than a couple of months, can put one at risk for various nutritional deficiencies. Besides vitamin B12, there is the potential for low levels of magnesium, iron, calcium, and others. These deficiencies may predispose not only to migraines but also to osteoporosis with bone fractures, dementia, cancer, birth defects, and infections.

Overall, supplements are safer than drugs. However, an herbal product can cause an allergic reaction and almost any supplement can upset your stomach. Supplements can interact with prescription medications. If you are taking any prescription drugs, consult with your doctor before taking supplements. Excessive amounts of certain supplements can be dangerous. You may want to follow the suggestions below and in the articles that are linked to the heading of each supplement.

33. Magnesium (8)

Magnesium deficiency is common in the general population. Up to half of migraine sufferers are deficient in magnesium. I have conducted and published research on the role of magnesium in migraines and have seen dramatic improvement from magnesium in many of my patients. For this reason, I strongly feel that every person with migraine headaches should try taking a magnesium supplement.

The American Headache Society and American Academy of Neurology guidelines consider magnesium supplementation to be "probably effective" for the prevention of migraine headaches. The reason magnesium is listed as only probably effective is that the clinical trials that have been done show inconsistent results. This is due to the poor design of these studies. For example, magnesium was given to all patients without regard to their magnesium blood level. Those who did not have a deficiency did not benefit from taking magnesium and they diluted positive results seen in those who were deficient.

Testing for magnesium deficiency is not straightforward. The most commonly done test is the serum magnesium level. Only 1% of the body's magnesium is found in the serum. Most of it is contained inside the cells. The uniqueness of our research was that we measured the more accurate ionized magnesium levels. This is a research test and is not available commercially. A test that is available and is more accurate than the serum level, is red blood cell (RBC) magnesium. Even with this test, the level should be at least in the middle of the normal range and not at the bottom of the range.

Ideally, magnesium should be obtained from foods like whole grains, dark leafy vegetables, avocados, legumes, and others. However, changing one's diet is not easy and sometimes is not sufficient to raise magnesium levels. This is due to poor absorption. The second-best choice is to take a supplement. I recommend starting with 400 mg of magnesium glycinate. Other magnesium salts can also help. For better absorption and to avoid diarrhea, take magnesium with food.

About 10%-20% of our patients who are deficient in magnesium either do not absorb magnesium – we check their RBC magnesium levels – or do not tolerate it and get diarrhea. Their migraines improve with a monthly intravenous infusion of magnesium.

Intravenous magnesium relieves acute migraine attacks in patients who are deficient in magnesium, according to a study we published in 1995 in the journal *Clinical Science*. An infusion not only stops an acute attack but also prevents migraines. We have hundreds of patients coming monthly for a five-minute infusion of one gram of magnesium sulfate. In some, a normal magnesium level is maintained after a few infusions and with an oral supplement. A small number of patients need to continue monthly infusions for years.

Research studies compared the absorption of various magnesium salts. Magnesium oxide was compared with chelated magnesium and a slow-release form of magnesium chloride. The study showed that all three types are absorbed equally well. Besides magnesium glycinate, other types of chelated magnesium (taurate, aspartate, gluconate, etc.) can be effective and well-tolerated. However, if one type of magnesium causes upset stomach or diarrhea, another one should be tried. Magnesium oxide, citrate, or carbonate can also help.

Magnesium has many benefits besides relieving migraines. It can possibly prevent Alzheimer's disease, reduce the size of a stroke, improve post-concussion syndrome, relieve fibromyalgia, palpitations, asthma, PMS, muscle cramps, "brain fog", and other symptoms. In a study of patients with mitral valve prolapse who had pronounced symptoms, 60% had a magnesium deficiency. Taking magnesium when compared to placebo significantly reduced all symptoms – weakness, chest pain, difficulty breathing, palpitations, and anxiety.

The only side effect of magnesium is an upset stomach or diarrhea. And the only people who should not take magnesium are those with serious kidney problems. It is safe and potentially beneficial to take a magnesium supplement during pregnancy.

34. Coenzyme Q10 (8)

Coenzyme Q_{10} (CoQ$_{10}$) is a necessary ingredient for the production of energy in every cell of the body. After magnesium, the deficiency of CoQ$_{10}$ is the second most common deficiency in migraine sufferers. One-third are deficient. This is according to a study by Dr. Andrew Hershey and his colleagues published in the journal *Headache*. They tested CoQ$_{10}$ levels in 1,550 children and adolescents and found 32.9% to be deficient. A study of such a large population makes the results reliable.

The researchers gave CoQ$_{10}$ only to children who were found to be deficient. Had they given CoQ$_{10}$ to all children, the study might have failed to show any benefit. This was the problem with most magnesium studies.

The children were given a daily dose of 1 to 3 mg/kg of CoQ$_{10}$. This produced significant improvement in CoQ$_{10}$ levels, the frequency of attacks, and the disability.

CoQ$_{10}$ deficiency is present in adults as well. This was shown in another study by a Swiss neurologist Dr. Peter Sandor and his colleagues. They compared 100 mg of CoQ$_{10}$ taken three times a day with placebo. Forty-eight percent of patients on CoQ$_{10}$ had a 50% drop in the number of migraine attacks compared to only 14% of patients on placebo.

The blood test for CoQ$_{10}$ can be expensive but may be covered by insurance. Just as with magnesium, vitamins D, and B$_{12}$, levels at the lower end of the normal range can indicate a deficiency. There is no harm in trying this supplement without first getting a blood test.

Side effects of CoQ_{10} are rare. Some people develop insomnia or have vivid dreams. Take this supplement in the morning. In my experience, 100 mg a day is usually sufficient.

The safety of CoQ_{10} was tested in doses of up to 900 mg. CoQ10 appears to be not only safe in pregnancy, but at 200 mg a day may prevent the development of pre-eclampsia.

35. Riboflavin (4)

Riboflavin or vitamin B_2, also facilitates the production of energy in cells. One Belgian study of riboflavin involved 55 migraine patients. They received a daily dose of either 400 mg of riboflavin or placebo for 3 months. Of those receiving riboflavin, 59% improved by at least 50% versus 15% on a placebo. However, the improvement occurred only in the third month. The results probably would have been much more impressive if riboflavin levels were measured and only those who were deficient were given riboflavin.

Don't become alarmed if your urine becomes bright yellow when you take riboflavin. There are no serious side effects from taking 400 mg of riboflavin. The daily recommended allowance, however, is only 1.4 mg. Doses lower than 400 mg daily are probably sufficient.

Despite its apparent safety, I would not recommend a 400 mg dose to pregnant women.

36. Vitamin D (4)

Many doctors, *The New York Times*, and other respected media outlets consider taking a vitamin D supplement of unproven benefit. However, solid scientific studies show the role of vitamin D deficiency in a wide variety of diseases. It has an effect on the development of delirium in hospitalized patients, the risk of major diseases and dying, COVID-19 infection, and probably migraines.

A 593-patient Mayo Clinic study reported increased severity of fibromyalgia in patients with vitamin D deficiency. Of these 593 patients, 122 or 21% had vitamin D deficiency. Patients with lower vitamin D levels also reported higher rates of anxiety and depression, and were more likely to be overweight.

Patients with multiple sclerosis (MS) whose vitamin D level is in the bottom quartile of the normal range are four times more likely to have a flare-up of their MS than those in the top quartile. Another MS study showed "...profound association of vitamin D levels with MRI measures of disease activity and progression". Those with vitamin D deficiency have a higher risk of developing Alzheimer's disease.

A group of Italian researchers examined 3 groups of subjects: 116 patients with chronic migraine, 44 patients with episodic migraine, and 100 non-headache controls. Ninety-two migraine patients had vitamin D insufficiency (borderline low levels), whereas 40 had vitamin D deficiency. There was a strong inverse correlation between vitamin D levels, the severity of attacks and migraine-related disability.

If you do get your vitamin D level tested, check what the actual result is. The normal range in most laboratories is from 30 to 100 ng/ml. However, if you are at the bottom of the normal range, you may be deficient. This predisposes one to a variety of medical conditions. Keep your level at least in the middle of this range.

37. Vitamin B12 and other B vitamins (4)

Vitamin B_{12} (cyanocobalamin) deficiency has been long suspected to play a role in the development of migraines. So far, it has not been directly linked to migraines.

An Iranian study published in the journal *Headache* compared vitamin B_{12} status in 70 migraine sufferers with 70 healthy people of similar age and sex. Serum levels of vitamin B_{12} were found to be significantly lower in migraine patients than in healthy subjects. Vitamin B_{12} levels are notoriously inaccurate. The authors also measured a more sensitive indicator of B_{12} deficiency, methylmalonic acid (MMA) level. MMA level goes up when vitamin B_{12} level goes down. Patients with the B_{12} levels in the highest quartile had an 80% lower chance of having migraines compared to those with levels in the bottom quartile. Patients in the highest quartile of MMA were five times more likely to have migraines.

Homocysteine is an amino acid that is normally present in the blood. An elevated level of homocysteine is another indirect indicator of vitamin B_{12} deficiency. In an Australian study, migraine sufferers with high homocysteine levels were given vitamins B_{12}, folic acid, and vitamin B_6. Their homocysteine levels dropped and migraine-related disability improved. Too much homocysteine can damage blood vessels. This could be in part responsible for the increased risk of strokes in patients with migraines with aura.

These studies show only a correlation between vitamin B_{12} levels and migraines. They do not prove that taking vitamin B_{12} relieves migraines.

Nevertheless, it makes sense to keep your level at least in the middle of the normal range since vitamin B_{12} is important for many brain functions. For example, multiple sclerosis patients with low B_{12} levels have a higher disability and vitamin B_{12} deficiency may predispose you to Alzheimer's disease.

Vegetarians and vegans are prone to vitamin B_{12} deficiency. The diabetes drug metformin, mentioned in the drug section of this book, can help with weight loss and possibly migraines but can cause B_{12} deficiency.

Most people who are deficient in vitamin B_{12} respond well to an oral supplement. A small proportion of patients do not seem to absorb vitamin B_{12} pills and feel better with regular (usually monthly) injections. These intramuscular injections can easily be self-administered. An intranasal form of vitamin B_{12} is also available but is expensive.

38. Zinc (2)

Edward Liveing felt that combining valerian with zinc made valerian more effective for the treatment of migraines.

Zinc deficiency was found in a small study of migraine patients by Turkish researchers. Supplementation with zinc relieved menstrual migraines in a Chinese study of 58 patients. While these two studies were of poor quality and published in obscure journals, a study showing that zinc relieves pain was published in one of the most prestigious journals, *Nature Neuroscience*.

Considering that zinc may also have a beneficial effect on our immune system, it may be worth trying a daily supplement of 25 mg of zinc.

39. Curcumin (3)

Curcurmin is effective in a rat model of migraine. Rats don't get migraines but researchers use rats to simulate brain changes seen in humans during a migraine attack.

When combined with omega-3 fatty acids, curcurmin was found to help human migraine sufferers as well. It has well documented anti-inflammatory properties and improves memory in healthy adults.

Curcumin is not well absorbed. Several companies have tried to improve its absorption using various methods. The memory study utilized Theracurmin, which is an ingredient in several brands of curcumin. Another brand, Longvida, also seems to be better absorbed.

40. Alpha-lipoic acid (3)

Alpha-lipoic acid (ALA), also known as thioctic acid, is present in every cell of the body. According to a study by Belgian researchers, a daily dose of 600 mg was significantly better than placebo in reducing the frequency of migraine attacks, headache days, and pain severity. No side effects were reported in this 44-patient study. However, a few of my patients have complained of an upset stomach, which is not surprising since it is an acid. This was a small study and it does not prove that ALA relieves migraines.

The use of this supplement is most proven in the treatment of painful peripheral neuropathies. ALA is available in Germany by prescription to treat diabetic peripheral neuropathy. This suggests that it may work for other painful neurological conditions such as migraine. ALA is being investigated as a treatment for multiple sclerosis, Alzheimer's disease, diabetes, strokes, and other conditions. The usual recommended dose is 300 mg twice a day.

41. Omega-3 fatty acids (3)

Omega-3 polyunsaturated fatty acids (PUFA) and omega-6 fatty acids are required for the body to produce pain-relieving and pain-enhancing substances.

Researchers at the University of North Carolina at Chapel Hill conducted a randomized, single-blind, parallel-group clinical trial, which was published in the journal Pain. Single-blind means that the doctor but not the patients know who is getting which treatment. The trial assessed the effects of changing the dietary intake of omega-3 and omega-6 fatty acids on chronic daily headaches.

After a 4-week baseline, patients undergoing usual care were randomized into one of two intensive, food-based 12-week dietary interventions. One group was given a high omega-3 plus low omega-6 diet and the second, a low omega-6 diet. The researchers measured headache-related disability using the Headache Impact Test (HIT-6). They also counted monthly headache days and the number of headache hours per day. The levels of omega-3 and omega-6 were measured in red blood cells. Of 67 enrolled patients, 56 completed the study.

Increasing omega-3 and lowering omega-6 produced significantly greater improvement in the HIT-6 score and the number of headache days per month compared to lowering omega-6. The first intervention also reduced the headache hours per day. The authors concluded that increasing omega-3 and reducing omega-6 fatty acids reduced headache pain and improved quality-of-life in chronic headache sufferers.

There are many other potential benefits of omega-3s. They help patients with coronary artery disease and diabetic nerve damage. Omega 3s can also protect against nerve damage by chemotherapy and prevent premature brain aging.

Eating fatty fish (that is low in mercury), such as salmon and sardines 2-3 times a week can be sufficient for general health. Those with coronary artery disease, migraines, and other conditions could benefit from a daily supplement.

There is little downside to taking an omega-3 supplement, as long as it is from a reputable store chain or a well-known brand. Cheaper brands can be contaminated by mercury.

42. Vitamin C (3)

Vitamin C or ascorbic acid (AA) deficiency appears to be more common in people with back pain, according to a study published in the journal *Pain* by Canadian researchers. AA is important for collagen formation. Collagen is one of the main ingredients of ligaments, tendons, and bones. Recent studies have reported that AA deficiency is common in the general population. The authors hypothesized that the "lack of AA contributes to poor collagen properties and back pain". The data from 4,742 individuals showed that low serum AA levels were associated with 1.5 times higher prevalence of neck pain and 1.3 times higher prevalence of low back pain. Low back pain with pain radiating to below the knee (sciatica) was also more common.

Neck pain is common in patients with migraine and tension-type headaches. This means that AA could also play a role in the treatment of headaches.

A case report published in *The New England Journal of Medicine* describes a 32-year-old man who controlled his migraine headaches with a daily dose of 6 grams of ascorbic acid for six years. He participated in a double-blind study in which he was given either AA or a placebo. At the end of 15 days, judging by the presence or absence of a headache, he correctly identified all the days on which he had received vitamin C and all the days when he was given a placebo.

A large 2020 study by Norwegian researchers confirmed that an elevated level of the inflammation marker, C-reactive protein (CRP) is associated with an increased risk of developing chronic migraine. A Japanese study of over 2,000 people showed that blood levels of vitamin C are inversely correlated with CRP levels. A review of 12 published studies of the effect of vitamin C on CRP showed that vitamin C lowers CRP levels.

AA is also important for the proliferation of stem cells. A study of 1,210 hospitalized patients showed that an intravenous infusion of AA in doses of 3–10 grams/day reduced the mortality of critically ill patients. AA plays a vital role in the functioning of the immune system and in inflammation. There are animal studies that suggest that AA is important in pain processing.

A wealth of information on AA is available on Oregon State University's Linus Pauling Institute website.

The recommended dietary allowance for AA is 75 mg for women and 90 mg for men. The Linus Pauling Institute suggests taking 400 mg a day, although many popular vitamin C supplements contain 1,000 mg or more. Taking 1,000 mg is safe. However, any amount of AA can cause heartburn or upset stomach because vitamin C is an acid.

It is possible to get enough vitamin C from food. Lemons and limes are rich in vitamin C but can upset the stomach. Though oranges and orange juice have too much sugar to eat in abundance, red peppers, kale, tomatoes, and strawberries are also good sources of vitamin C.

43. Vitamin E (2)

A single double-blind placebo-controlled trial of 400 units of vitamin E in 72 women showed it to be effective in treating menstrual migraines.

A meta-analysis of 12 published trials showed that vitamin E (αtocopherol or γtocopherol) lowers the level of an inflammation marker C-reactive protein (CRP). As mentioned in the section on vitamin C, an elevated CRP level can increase the risk of developing chronic migraine.

44. Melatonin (3)

Melatonin is a hormone produced by the pineal gland located in the brain. The release of melatonin helps us fall asleep. Melatonin supplements have been used to treat insomnia. The results of clinical trials, however, are contradictory. This may be because a wide variety of doses have been used. One study suggests that 3 mg of melatonin – a common dose sold in stores – is less effective than 0.3 mg. I usually recommend 0.3 mg (300 mcg) for both insomnia and jet lag.

Melatonin has been tested for the prevention and acute treatment of migraines.

Melatonin was not effective in a study by Norwegian doctors. They gave 2 mg of extended-release melatonin every night for 8 weeks to 46 migraine sufferers. All 46 also received 8 weeks of placebo in a double-blind crossover trial. Migraine frequency did improve from an average of 4.2 a month to 2.8 in both the melatonin and the placebo groups.

Another blinded trial was done in Brazil by Dr. Mario Peres and his colleagues. It compared 3 mg of immediate-release melatonin with a placebo and with 25 mg of amitriptyline. The study involved 196 patients. The number of headache days dropped by 2.7 days in the melatonin group, 2.2 for amitriptyline, and 1.2 for placebo. Melatonin significantly reduced headache frequency compared to placebo. Amitriptyline did not. Not surprisingly, melatonin was much better tolerated than amitriptyline. Considering its safety and very low cost, it is worth considering a trial of 3 mg of melatonin daily for the prevention of migraine headaches.

It is possible that, unlike with insomnia, a higher dose is more effective for the prevention of migraines. And, the immediate-release form could be more effective than the sustained-release one.

Melatonin may be effective as an acute treatment for pediatric migraine, according to a study conducted by Dr. Amy Gelfand and her colleagues at UCSF. This was an 84-patient trial, although only 46 children completed it. Both low and high doses of melatonin were associated with pain reduction. Higher dose and napping after treatment predicted greater benefit. The benefit was likely an indirect one – melatonin helped children fall asleep. And sleep, very often in children but also in some adults, can relieve a migraine attack.

Herbal treatments

45. Boswellia/Gliacin (4)

Boswellia or Indian frankincense (*Boswellia serrata*) has been popular for the treatment of joint pains. A double-blind, crossover study by Indian researchers showed that it is effective for the treatment of osteoarthritis of the knee.

Boswellia has long been used to relieve migraines as well. However, there are no scientific articles to support this observation.

A study published in the journal *Cephalalgia* by Christian Lampl and his colleagues describes four patients with chronic cluster headaches whose headaches improved after taking Boswellia extract. The dose of Boswellia was 350 to 700 mg three times a day. All four of these patients had failed at least three standard preventive medications for cluster headaches – verapamil, topiramate, and lithium. Surprisingly, an herbal remedy helped this very painful type of headache.

Dr. Eric Eross reported that Boswellia extract, gliacin, helped indomethacin-responsive headaches. These headaches are described at the end of the book. Indomethacin is a strong non-steroidal anti-inflammatory medication, but it also tends to have strong gastrointestinal side effects. Of the 27 patients with these types of headaches who were given Boswellia, 21 improved. The starting dose was 250 mg three times a day. The dose was increased as needed, although it is not clear what the highest dose was.

Boswellia does not have any toxic ingredients and is safe to consume in any form.

46. Feverfew (4)

Feverfew (*tanacetum parthenium*) is one of the oldest herbal remedies for the treatment of migraine headaches. The first-century Greek physician Pedanius Dioscorides prescribed feverfew for "all hot inflammations". Feverfew is a member of the daisy family. All of the above-ground parts of the plants are safe to eat. It is usually consumed as dried leaves or tea made of dried flowers. It has been used for the treatment of fevers, rheumatoid arthritis, stomach aches, toothaches, insect bites, psoriasis, allergies, asthma, tinnitus, dizziness, nausea, vomiting, infertility, and other problems.

We have some scientific evidence for the effectiveness of feverfew in the prevention of migraine headaches. Five clinical trials have been published.

British researchers conducted a study of feverfew in 60 migraine patients. Half of them received feverfew and the other half, placebo. After four months, the treatment was switched (so-called crossover study). Patients in the feverfew group had 4.7 fewer attacks per month. Taking a placebo resulted in 3.6 fewer attacks. Feverfew also reduced the severity of nausea and vomiting of migraines.

A <u>more rigorous study by German researchers</u> enrolled 170 migraineurs. Eighty-nine were given an extract of feverfew and 81, a placebo. The number of monthly migraine attacks dropped by 1.9 in the feverfew group and by 1.3 attacks in the placebo group. There was also a difference in the global assessment of efficacy.

Feverfew occasionally causes mouth sores. Like any herbal product, feverfew can cause an upset stomach or an allergic reaction.

Another issue that applies to all herbal products is that every manufacturer processes the plant differently. In some cases, the product contains little or no active ingredients. You should buy products made by large reputable manufacturers. Feverfew can also be grown in a pot or planted in a garden.

47. Valerian (3)

For centuries, the root of valerian (*Valeriana officinalis*) has been a popular remedy for anxiety, insomnia, and migraines. Edward Liveing recommended valerian for the treatment of migraines in a book he wrote in 1873. Liveing quotes from a book published in 1758 by Dr. J. Fordyce. Fordyce had great success in treating his own migraines with large doses of valerian. As mentioned above, Liveing felt that a combination of valerian and zinc was more effective than valerian alone.

Valerian was reported <u>to help migraines</u> in two <u>small studies</u>. It is most often used for anxiety and insomnia that are common in people with migraines.

Valerian is sold in tablets, capsules, as tea, and tincture.

48. Butterbur (4)

The New York Headache Center was one of the three clinics that participated in a 245-patient, double-blind, placebo-controlled trial of butterbur. The German manufacturer of the butterbur product, Petadolex, sponsored this study. The trial showed that 150 mg of butterbur is more effective in preventing migraine headaches than the placebo. <u>The results were published in a leading neurological journal,</u> *Neurology.* Following this study, the American Academy of Neurology endorsed the use of butterbur for the prevention of migraine headaches. A few years later, they withdrew this endorsement.

Germany regulates supplements as strictly as drugs. To receive approval, every supplement has to undergo safety studies. This is particularly crucial for butterbur products. Raw butterbur is highly toxic to the liver, can cause cancer, and birth defects.

When our butterbur manufacturer changed the extraction and purification process, the German regulatory agency, The Federal Institute for Drugs and Medical Devices, asked to repeat all of the safety studies. These studies are expensive and the manufacturer decided not to repeat them. Butterbur is no longer sold in Germany but is still produced there for sale in the US. The FDA inspected the manufacturing plant in Germany and found it to be compliant with all of the FDA's requirements.

The brand Petadolex is expensive – about $60 a month – and I am concerned that some people may decide to buy a cheaper brand of butterbur. Some of them cost $5 for a month's supply. Since the cheaper products can be dangerous, I advise using only the brand Petadolex.

49. Ginger (3)

Ginger is not only a popular spice but a truly remarkable medicinal plant. Ginger has proven anti-inflammatory properties. This may be responsible for its beneficial effect in migraine patients. Ginger may be effective for seasickness, morning sickness of pregnancy, and for nausea of migraine.

A study published in the journal of the International Headache Society, *Cephalalgia*, examined the effect of ginger as an add-on to intravenous pain medication.

This was a double-blind placebo-controlled randomized clinical trial performed in the emergency room of a general hospital in Brazil. Sixty adults with migraines with or without aura were included in this study. Thirty participants were given 400 mg of ginger extract (5% active ingredient) and thirty, placebo. This was in addition to 100 mg of intravenous ketoprofen. Ketoprofen is not available in the US. It is similar to ketorolac which is widely used in the US emergency rooms. Pain severity, functional status, migraine symptoms, and treatment satisfaction were recorded.

Patients treated with ginger showed significantly better pain relief after one, one and a half, and two hours. Ginger also significantly improved functional status and overall satisfaction.

Another double-blind study by Iranian doctors involved 100 patients. It compared the efficacy of ginger with sumatriptan in the treatment of an acute migraine attack. Patient satisfaction and their willingness to continue treatment were evaluated after 1 month following the initial treatment. Two hours after using either drug, the mean headache severity significantly decreased. The efficacy of ginger and sumatriptan was similar. The adverse effects of ginger were less than those of sumatriptan. Patient satisfaction was similar in both groups.

Because ginger has anti-inflammatory properties, it is possible that taking it daily may also prevent migraines. Preventive trials have not been conducted.

I usually recommend a daily dose of 500 mg of dried ginger in capsules. Eating fresh ginger or using it in cooking is healthful but is less likely to provide a sufficiently high amount to have an impact on migraine.

50. Homeopathic remedies (2)

Homeopathy uses infinitesimally small amounts of herbal products to treat many medical conditions. Several scientific studies have shown that homeopathy is not much better than a placebo. But this is not so bad. The placebo in some controlled migraine trials helps as many as 50% of trial participants. If you consider that homeopathic remedies are inexpensive and safe, this could be a good and ethical form of placebo. Giving a plain placebo such as a sugar pill is considered unethical.

One fascinating study of placebo by Harvard researchers showed that even when people know that they are taking a placebo, their symptoms improve.

So, go ahead and try homeopathy to treat your migraines. I sometimes recommend homeopathic remedies to patients who have a strong compulsion to take medicine. They take prescription or non-prescription drugs very frequently. The reason is the fear of the headache becoming uncontrollable. Most pharmacies in the US carry a range of homeopathic remedies and there is always at least one product for the treatment of headaches or migraines.

51. Probiotics (2)

Our body is made up of about 30 trillion cells but we also contain 100 trillion bacterial cells. It is not surprising that we cannot survive without these bacteria and having the wrong balance of different types of bacteria can make us sick. You can read about this remarkable symbiotic relationship in a fascinating book by Ed Yong, *I Contain Multitudes: The Microbes Within Us and a Grander View of Life.*

Many migraine sufferers have intestinal problems, such as irritable bowel syndrome (IBS), constipation, sensitivity to gluten, dairy, and other types of foods. Nausea and vomiting and gastric stasis (lack of normal propulsive movement) are common during a migraine attack. This suggests a close relationship between the gut and migraines.

Probiotics are supplements that contain various types of bacteria. Probiotics are popular for the treatment of different digestive problems, allergic conditions, and metabolic problems.

Bio-Kult is a probiotic that contains 14 different strains of bacteria. It was tested for the prevention of migraine headaches in a double-blind placebo-controlled trial. The results were published in *Cephalalgia*. The Iranian researchers enrolled 100 patients and placed half of them into the placebo group and the other half into the probiotic group. Forty-three patients in the active group and 36 in the placebo group completed the trial.

After two months of treatment, the mean frequency of migraine attacks and their severity were significantly reduced in the probiotic group. This did not happen in the placebo group. There was also a significant reduction in the number of acute migraine medications taken by patients in the probiotic group.

The study had a high dropout rate. This makes it difficult to assess the validity of the results. However, considering its safety and reasonable cost, it may be worth trying. Bio-Kult is manufactured in the UK, which suggests that it is of good quality.

For patients with gastrointestinal problems, I also recommend trying probiotics that contain other types of bacteria. Some of the more popular US brands include Florastor, Culturelle, Align, and Nature's Way Fortify. Try one for a couple of months and if there is no change, try another one. You never know which bacteria you may be lacking.

52. CBD / cannabis (4)

Medical marijuana (MM) is legal in many states, including the state of New York. MM does not help the majority of my patients. A significant minority, however, finds it helpful. The benefits may include relief of pain, nausea, anxiety, and improved sleep.

An observational study of 121 migraine patients in Colorado showed that 40% found MM beneficial. Another study was done at a headache clinic in the state of Washington. The researchers interviewed 4,386 new patients about their use of marijuana. Only 437, or 10% tried marijuana. About 60% of those who tried it found it helpful. Both studies found that marijuana rarely completely relieves an acute migraine. It was more effective for the prevention of attacks, the reduction of pain severity, and nausea.

Various ratios of two main ingredients in MM, tetrahydrocannabinol (THC) and cannabidiol (CBD) produce different effects. Often, neither one alone is as effective as a combination of the two. Raphael Mechoulam, a Hebrew University chemist who discovered THC, calls this the entourage effect.

We still don't fully understand how MM works, in what combination of ingredients, and for what types of pain.

Releaf is a smartphone app that is used to record various symptoms people treat with marijuana. It also tracks the type of product people use and how they use it. The maker of the app has published the results of marijuana treatment in 699 migraine and headache patients. Ninety-four percent of users had symptom relief within two hours. This high response rate is not surprising – those for whom marijuana did not help would not continue taking it and they would not use the app. The average symptom intensity reduction was 3.3 points on a 0–10 scale. Men had greater relief than women. Users younger than 35 had greater relief than older users. Products containing 10% or more of THC provided the best symptom relief. Women and younger users had greater symptom relief from *Cannabis indica* strain than from *Cannabis sativa* or mixtures of strains.

A few of my patients take MM daily for the prevention of migraine attacks. The majority use it as needed, whenever an attack occurs. MM often relieves pain, nausea, or migraine-induced anxiety. Some patients find that it helps them to go to sleep and when they wake up, the headache is gone. A few patients have told me that they take it regularly for insomnia. It works better than prescription sleep medicines and does not cause side effects. The calming effect of MM is useful to treat anxiety, including anticipatory anxiety. Anticipatory anxiety is caused by the fear of the next often unpredictable migraine attack.

One of the advantages of using MM over other marijuana products is the consistent composition and quality of the ingredients. This consistency sometimes applies only to a specific manufacturer. People find that products from one dispensary are more effective than from another even when using products with the same concentration of THC and CBD. This can be explained by the fact that all MM products contain other supposedly inactive ingredients. These ingredients may very well be active and have positive or negative effects.

It is legal to buy CBD oil made from hemp without a doctor's prescription. It can be purchased in stores as well as online. For many, CBD works well to relieve pain, nausea, and symptoms of inflammation.

Some patients take low-THC/high-CBD products during the day to avoid euphoric and cognitive effects. At night they might take a high-THC/low-CD mixture.

Vaping MM provides the fastest effect. For prevention, taking a tablet or a tincture can be more convenient.

The main problem with smoking marijuana instead of taking MM by mouth is that smoke from the burning plant causes lung damage. Vaping has also been reported to cause lung damage, but never from a regulated medical marijuana product.

Aromatherapy

53. Peppermint (2)

Peppermint has been used for centuries internally, topically, and as aromatherapy. In a study of 128 pregnant women, 64 received peppermint oil inhalation and 64 did not. The study showed that peppermint reduces pain and anxiety in the first stage of labor. Peppermint oil taken by mouth is proven to relieve the pain of IBS, a condition that is more common in migraine sufferers. A rigorous scientific study of the effect of peppermint oil on pain was done by Dr. Hartmut Göbel, a headache and pain specialist in Kiel, Germany. He compared peppermint and eucalyptus oil preparations on various neurophysiological and experimental pain parameters. It was a double-blind, placebo-controlled, randomized cross-over trial in 32 healthy subjects. He discovered that a combination of peppermint and eucalyptus oil enhanced cognitive abilities, had muscle-relaxing and mentally-relaxing effects. Only peppermint oil had a pain-relieving effect.

54. Lavender (2)

Smelling lavender oil also relieves pain. This was shown in several clinical studies in healthy volunteers, patients with postoperative pain, procedural (needle insertion) pain, and post-tonsillectomy pain in children.

It is unlikely that aromatherapy alone will stop a severe migraine attack. However, it may provide additional relief when combined with other measures or medications. Because migraines can be triggered by odors, one strategy I recommend is carrying a small vial of essential oils of peppermint or lavender to block the noxious smells. Migrastick is a popular brand sold in most pharmacies. It combines peppermint and lavender oils in a small glass vial topped with a rollerball.

Electric stimulation

55. Transcranial direct current stimulation* (3)

Transcranial direct current stimulation (tDCS) is performed by applying two electrodes to the scalp. These electrodes are connected to a battery-operated device. tDCS has been shown to alter brain connectivity, improves memory, relieve depression, and produce other brain effects. Several studies of tDCS suggest that it may be effective for the treatment of migraines, including refractory or difficult to treat ones. A review of tDCS for the treatment of migraine headaches identifies problems with this potentially effective therapy. The majority of studies were pilot studies that were not blinded and performed in a small number of patients. Another problem was a great variation in stimulation duration, intensity, and electrode placement. The number of stimulation sessions also differed across studies (3–22 sessions).

Most published studies required patients to visit the doctor's office for each treatment. A much more promising, practical, and probably more effective approach is having patients apply TDCs daily at home. Such devices have been approved and are sold in Europe for the treatment of pain and depression. They lack such approval in the US but because they are considered safe, you can buy them without a prescription in the US as well.

56. Transcutaneous electric nerve stimulation* (4)

Transcutaneous electric nerve stimulation (TENS) also involves attaching electrodes that are connected to a small battery-operated device. The current, however, is alternating and the electrodes are applied to the skin of the forehead or the body. TENS is an old and proven method for the treatment of musculoskeletal pain. It is widely used in physical therapy. It also seems to be effective for the treatment of migraines.

One issue with TENS is that you need to figure out the optimal frequency and strength of stimulation. This can take time and requires patience.

A group of Chinese doctors compared TENS over the occipital nerves (the nerves at the back of the head) with the preventive drug topiramate. They have found that applying TENS at 100 Hz frequency of stimulation daily for 30 minutes was as effective as topiramate.

Cefaly is a TENS device that is applied to the forehead. It is cleared by the FDA for the acute and preventive treatment of migraines. The approval was based on a 67-patient double-blind study. TENS devices do not require large clinical trials that are demanded by the FDA for drugs. Some of my patients find it effective. They mostly use it for the acute treatment of migraine attacks. Cefaly is safe and easy to use. Not inexpensive, its cost is approximately four hundred dollars. A basic TENS unit with sticky electrodes and wires costs as little as $50 but is more awkward to apply.

Nerivio is a device approved by the FDA for the acute treatment of migraine attacks. It works differently than other TENS units because it involves stimulation of a remote site to produce central or brain effects. Also, the frequency of stimulation fluctuates throughout the session. Nerivio is applied to the upper arm and is controlled by a smartphone app.

Nerivio was proven to be effective in a double-blind, sham-controlled study of 252 adults with migraine headaches. It was applied for 45 minutes after the onset of migraine. The strength of the current was gradually increased to strong but non-painful intensity. True stimulation was more effective than sham stimulation in achieving pain relief, pain-free state, and relief of the most bothersome symptom such as nausea, sensitivity to light or noise 2 hours after treatment. The pain relief and pain-free superiority of the true treatment was sustained for 48 hours. The treatment was well tolerated with only a few patients reporting local irritation.

Nerivio is a disposable device that provides 12 treatments. Each device costs $99 but some insurance plans will pay for it.

57. Non-invasive vagus nerve stimulation* (3)

Vagus nerve is a nerve in the neck that connects the brain to most internal organs. Vagus nerve stimulation (VNS) can be done by applying an electrode to the skin of the neck or with an electrode surgically implanted and wrapped around the nerve. The implantable device is approved by the FDA for the treatment of depression and epilepsy when these conditions do not respond to medications.

Because antidepressant and anti-epilepsy medications help migraines, I treated four chronic migraine patients and two cluster headache patients with an implanted VNS device. Headaches in these patients did not respond to many different types of treatments. Two of the four chronic migraine patients and both cluster patients obtained good relief. <u>The description of these patients and their treatment was published in 2005 in the journal *Cephalalgia*</u>.

This publication spurred the development of <u>gammaCore</u>. This is a hand-held device that is used to stimulate the vagus nerve through the skin. I participated in one of the earliest studies of this device <u>and the results were encouraging</u>.

After a series of studies, gammaCore received approval from the FDA for the acute treatment of pain associated with migraine and cluster headaches. It is also approved for the preventive treatment of migraines and cluster headaches.

gammaCore is expensive and most insurance companies do not cover this or any other electric stimulation device.

58. Transcranial magnetic stimulation* (3)

Transcranial magnetic stimulation (TMS) involves stimulation of the brain with a magnetic field. TMS has been researched for over 30 years. It is used to study the brain and is being explored to treat depression, Parkinson's disease, stroke, pain, and other brain disorders.

The FDA approved <u>eNeura Transcranial Magnetic Stimulator</u> for the acute and prophylactic treatment of migraine headaches with aura in adults and adolescents. Several clinical trials <u>showed that if used at the time of aura, it will provide relief of pain that follows the aura</u>. Another <u>study showed that this device may be also effective for the prevention of migraine attacks</u>.

Adverse events reported during these studies were rare. Patients must not use the TMS device if they have any metal in the head, neck, or upper body or if they have an active implanted medical device such as a pacemaker or deep brain stimulator. It should not be used in patients with suspected or diagnosed epilepsy, personal or family history of seizures.

The device is expensive, bulky, and inconvenient to carry around. It is useful for people who have severe disabling migraines that do not respond to other treatments.

In August of 2020 the manufacturer of this device filed for bankruptcy. It is not clear if the product will ever return to the market.

59. Implanted electrical stimulators (1)

Doctors have tried stimulating the nervous system with electric current since such current became available. They continue to try to stimulate it through the surface of the skin and by implanting wires next to the nerve, spinal cord, and even inside the brain. Blinded studies are hard to do with implanted devices because people feel the electric current, so they know if they are getting it or not.

Occipital nerve blocks described below can stop a migraine attack. This has led to many attempts to prevent migraines by electrically stimulating these nerves using implantable devices. Studies of this treatment tend to be positive, but the trials are small and not convincing. I have never referred a patient for an occipital nerve stimulator. Surgery has complications and is expensive, migraines may improve on their own, and many of the 150 other approaches can be tried first.

Doctors also implant electrodes that stimulate the supraorbital nerve, which is located in the forehead. Combined stimulation of both the occipital and supraorbital nerves in seven patients was better than the stimulation of either one by itself.

Injections and blocks

60. OnabotulinumtoxinA* (8)

In the early 1990s, I was one of the first neurologists to start injecting onabotulinumtoxinA (Botox) for the treatment of migraine headaches. Many of my colleagues were incredulous. They could not believe that a treatment directed at the superficial nerves and muscles would help a brain disorder such as migraine. At first, we thought that relaxing tight muscles around the scalp was responsible for the relief that many patients reported. Since then, scientists have discovered that Botox stops nerve endings in the scalp from sending pain messages to the brain. This disrupts the vicious cycle that indeed begins in the brain but requires a response from the peripheral nerve endings.

My most dramatic result from Botox injections occurred in a 76-year-old woman. She had been suffering from migraines for 60 years and for the previous 20 years they were occurring daily. She was referred by an experienced neurologist who ran out of options in trying to help her. My first thought was that after 60 years of relentless migraines her brain circuits were burnt-in and nothing could break the vicious cycle of pain. Three months after her first Botox treatment she called to report that this was the first time in her life that she had three months without a single migraine.

More than 250 doctors from around the world have visited our clinic for training in Botox injections. We've participated in one of the <u>pivotal trials that led to the approval of Botox for the treatment of chronic migraines.</u> I have <u>written extensively</u> on <u>my blog</u>, <u>in articles</u>, and in <u>book chapters. One of the chapters appeared in the book on headaches in the 174-volume (!)</u> *Handbook of Clinical Neurology*.

Despite all of my and my colleagues' efforts, as well as promotions by the manufacturer, Botox remains highly underutilized. These are some possible explanations.

1. Botox is expensive and many insurance companies make it difficult for patients to get it.

2. There are several million chronic migraine sufferers who could benefit from Botox but only a few thousand neurologists who can administer it.

3. Chronic migraines are often misdiagnosed as episodic migraines. This is important because insurers will cover Botox only for chronic migraines. Botox, however, is also highly effective for patients with episodic migraines – patients who have fewer than 15 headache days each month. <u>The experts are proposing changing the definition of chronic migraine to having 8 or more migraine days each month.</u>

4. Some patients are afraid of Botox because it is a poison. It is true that by weight, it is the deadliest poison known to man. However, it is very

safe because the amount injected is infinitesimally small. It is measured in nanograms. Also, the drug remains at the site of injection and does not spread throughout the body. This is why Botox is safer than any drug taken by mouth.

In summary, if you have headaches on more than half of the days and you've tried two preventive drugs and non-drug treatments, find a doctor who knows how to give Botox injections. Botox is more effective and safer than preventive medications. It does not affect your liver, kidneys, brain, or any other organ. If you are concerned about the pain of injections and want to see how the procedure is done, watch YouTube videos of two of my patients who agreed to have their injections filmed.

Common avoidable problems with Botox:

1. One of the most common problems is that doctors use the standard FDA-approved protocol without adjusting the dose. One of my patients was an 83-year-old woman with chronic migraines. She had done exceptionally well with Botox injections for over 16 years. She moved to Florida and had Botox injections given by a local doctor. I provided her with a copy of the injection sites and the total dose, which was one-third of the standard amount. Her Florida neurologist insisted on giving her 31 injections with 155 units, including in the areas where she never had pain. As a result, she developed drooping of her eyelids, pain, and weakness of her neck. It defies common sense to give the same amount of Botox to a 90-lb person whose headaches are limited to the forehead as a 180-lb person with pain all around the head, neck, and shoulders.

2. Strict adherence to the protocol also prevents many doctors from giving additional injections for clenching and grinding of the teeth, or TMJ syndrome. TMJ syndrome often worsens migraines. Injecting Botox into the chewing muscles at the corner of the lower jaw can stop clenching and grinding. Adding these injections provides better relief of migraines than the standard protocol.

3. Other patients may need additional injections into the scalp or upper back, depending on where the pain is felt.

4. Botox is given every 12 weeks. This works well for many patients. However, about a quarter of my migraine patients find that the effect of Botox does not last 12 weeks. In some, it lasts for only 10-11 weeks, and in a small number of patients, 8-9 weeks. Some insurance companies allow Botox to be administered earlier than 12 weeks, but

many do not. Having a week or two of worsening migraines can eliminate the cumulative effect we see with repeated treatments. If given on time, each subsequent Botox treatment provides better relief than the previous one. This may not happen if the headaches worsen before the next scheduled treatment.

5.   Doctors from the Ochsner Neuroscience Institute reported that 44% of their patients had the duration of effect less than 12 weeks. Drs. Masters-Israilov and Robbins reported that out of 143 patients, Botox produced relief for less than 12 weeks in 90 (63%). In some of their patients, the effect lasted less than 8 weeks. In most, wearing off occurred in the last 2-4 weeks. Their study suggested that wearing off is less likely to occur with higher doses of Botox. Fortunately, a vial of Botox contains 200 units. This allows us to give doses higher than 155 units to most patients. The authors reported using nerve blocks, injections of ketorolac, and steroid medications to tie patients over until their next Botox treatment.

6.   For most people, the cosmetic effect of Botox is an added benefit. A bad cosmetic outcome, however, can happen. This is not trivial because Botox injections can make you look strange. Some people develop a surprised or sinister look because the ends of their eyebrows are always lifted. This can be avoided by injecting a small amount of Botox into the appropriate muscles above the ends of the eyebrows. Many cosmetic problems can be corrected with a few additional small injections. Drooping of the eyelids can be avoided with proper injection technique. If this does happen, apraclonidine 0.5% eye drops used for glaucoma can help lift the eyelids. If eye drops are ineffective or cause side effects, a cosmetic double-sided tape that is specifically used to lift droopy eyelids can help.

7.   Very thin needles can minimize bruising and pain. A 30-gauge needle is used most often, however, an even thinner, 33-gauge needle is also available but is rarely used. A higher number indicates a thinner needle.

8.   Cost is the only major issue with Botox injections. However, since it is FDA-approved, it is covered by almost all insurance companies. Botox relieves migraine headaches to various degrees in 70% of migraine sufferers. A study published by Dr. John Rothrock and his colleagues at the University of Nevada in the journal Headache indicates that Botox is not only clinically effective but is also cost-effective.

Researchers from the Renown Neurosciences Institute in Reno, Nevada analyzed data from 230 chronic migraine sufferers who did not respond to two or more prophylactic drugs and were given Botox injections. Botox was given twice, three months apart. Compared with the 6 months before Botox, there were 55% fewer emergency room visits, 59% fewer urgent care visits, and 57% fewer admissions to the hospital. In those 6 months, the savings amounted to half of the cost of Botox treatments. Considering that improvement tends to get more pronounced with each subsequent Botox treatment, it is likely that the cost savings grow with additional treatments.

61. Nerve blocks (4)

Nerve blocks consist of injecting a drug such as lidocaine or bupivacaine to numb the nerves around the scalp. The most commonly blocked nerves are occipital, which are in the back of the head. We also block supraorbital (forehead) and temporal (temples) nerves. Your head will feel numb for a few hours from these shots. For many people, this stops the attack of migraine. There is some evidence that weekly nerve blocks can prevent migraine attacks. Patients who respond well to nerve blocks but not other treatments may want to consider having temporary destruction of the nerves. This is done using heat from a radiofrequency probe, or so-called radiofrequency ablation.

Nerve blocks are useful for people who do not respond to medications or have contraindications to taking drugs such as triptans, and pregnant women who prefer to avoid taking medications.

Weekly nerve blocks can also help patients who respond well to Botox injections, but in whom the effect lasts less than 12 weeks and the insurer does not allow more frequent injections.

62. Sphenopalatine ganglion blocks (3)

The sphenopalatine ganglion (SPG) is a collection of nerve cells underneath the skull and behind your nasal cavity. These cells have a wide network of connections and numbing these cells with a local anesthetic such as bupivacaine seems to help migraine headaches, according to a study by Dr. Roger Cady, Joel Saper, and their colleagues. The procedure involves the insertion of a thin plastic catheter through each nostril to the area near the ganglion. It is not painful and can be effective when nerve blocks don't work. Catheters for this procedure are only made by two small companies and are relatively expensive.

Migraine surgery

63. Contact point surgery (3)

A severely deviated nasal septum that results in a "contact point" can be a migraine trigger. The septum divides the left and the right side of the nose. It is made of cartilage in the front of the nose and bone in the back. If the bony part of the septum is very deviated, which often happens from an injury, it sometimes touches the side of the nose. This creates a contact point between the septum and the side wall of the nose. If headaches are constant, the constant pressure of the contact point would explain the pain. However, sometimes people with intermittent migraine attacks respond as well. Here is a theory of how a contact point could cause intermittent migraines: Intermittent congestion and swelling of the mucous lining of the nasal cavity increases the pressure at the contact point and triggers a headache. The swelling can be caused by nasal congestion due to allergies, red wine, exercise, and possibly other migraine triggers.

Surgical removal of this contact point can improve your migraines. It is possible to predict who may respond to contact point surgery. The doctor can spray a local anesthetic, such as lidocaine, around the contact point during a migraine attack and if the pain goes away, then surgery is more likely to help. Patients can also try putting lidocaine drops into their nose during an attack.

64. Denervation surgery (3)

Surgery for refractory migraine headaches was developed by Dr. Bahman Guyuron. Good results have been reported in 68% to 95% of patients. This surgery involves cutting or freeing up nerves in the scalp that appear to be responsible for triggering migraines. Some surgeons use a laparoscopic technique, which involves making only a few small incisions. Others perform this surgery through conventional incisions.

Drs. Gfrerer, Maman, and their colleagues at the Massachusetts General Hospital in Boston published their results in a paper *Non-Endoscopic Deactivation of Nerve Triggers in Migraine Headache Patients: Surgical Technique and Outcomes.* The authors argue that endoscopic techniques may not be appropriate in many cases. Some surgeons have little experience or limited access to the endoscope. In some patients, this technique is not practical because the nerves could run in an unusual pattern. This would make them hard to find through a small incision. This study involved 43 consecutive procedures in 35 patients. All patients completed questionnaires before and 12 months after the surgery. The overall positive response rate was 91%. Total elimination of migraine headaches was reported in 51%, greater than 80% resolution of symptoms in 21%, and 28% had resolution between 50-80%. No improvement was reported after 9% of procedures. There were no serious adverse events.

The authors concluded that non-endoscopic surgery was a safe and effective treatment in select migraine headache patients.

Because the placebo response to surgery is very high, most headache experts agree that until proven effective in large controlled studies, surgery should only be done as part of a large controlled trial. However, even with surgery, the placebo response is rarely 90% and the effect rarely lasts 12 months. Considering these facts, that this study was done at a reputable institution, and that their patients had refractory migraines (i.e. they did not respond to conventional therapy, including Botox), surgery may be truly effective for some patients.

Mind-body

For this is the great error of our day ... that physicians separate the soul from the body.

—Plato

To most people, it is obvious that stress is a major trigger for headaches. Many patients cannot understand why they have no migraines during stressful times but when the stress is over, they get a severe attack. For some, it happens every weekend, on vacations, or just when they can take a break from the hectic pace of their lives. This is probably because some people can keep their migraines under control when they have to perform. As soon as they can relax, their control relaxes too. I tell such patients that this means that they can learn to control their migraines all the time.

65. Biofeedback/neurofeedback (8)

Biofeedback is an excellent preventive treatment for migraine headaches. Its efficacy is proven in dozens of rigorous studies. A meta-analysis of 55 such studies showed a consistently high efficacy. Children tend to learn biofeedback with greater ease than adults. They often need only 4 or 5 sessions instead of the usual 10 or more. Biofeedback is a way to learn to relax and stay relaxed under pressure. The person learning biofeedback is connected to a computer by a probe that measures the body's temperature or muscle tension. In the case of neurofeedback, patients monitor their brain waves. This information is displayed on a screen, which helps you learn how to relax your body. Biofeedback is taught by a psychologist, a nurse, or another trained professional.

Studies show that self-taught <u>relaxation training can be as effective as biofeedback</u>. You may be skeptical about the efficacy of biofeedback or relaxation training. There is a simple explanation of how it works. If you stop for a minute or even for a few seconds to take an inventory of neck, facial, and other muscles and take a few deep breaths, your tension will go down just a little. If you repeat this one-minute exercise every hour or two, at the end of the day you will avoid the build-up of tension, knots in your shoulders and your neck, and migraine. Eventually, this exercise becomes subconscious as you automatically monitor your body. Whenever you feel tense, finding yourself frowning, holding shoulders up, or holding your breath, you stop doing that without a pause.

Slow breathing which is a part of most relaxation exercises has been shown to have a <u>pain-relieving effect in healthy volunteers.</u>

Developed by the American physician Edmund Jacobson in the 1920s, progressive relaxation is a simple method of relaxing the muscles that can be performed without any training. Through tensing and relaxing your muscles, one by one, you teach your mind and body a way of recognizing how stress creates muscle tension and how to release it.

Here is an example of a progressive relaxation exercise (adapted from *The Headache Alternative: A Neurologist's Guide to Drug-Free Relief,* A. Mauskop and M. A. Brill, Dell 1997):

1. Get comfortable. Wear loose clothing, remove your shoes. Make sure you are neither too warm or cold. Find a quiet room where you won't be distracted for 15 minutes.

2. Sit in a comfortable chair, or lie down on the ground on your back, using an exercise mat or soft carpet.

3. Take a few deep relaxing breaths.

4. Tense all of the muscles in your body, from head to toe. Hold the tension for several seconds. Let your mind feel the sensation of this tension.

5. Holding onto the tension, inhale deeply, and hold your breath for several seconds. Let your mind and body register the sensation of this tension.

6. Exhale slowly as you let the tension go. Let your mind and body register the sensation of this relaxation.

Now, work on individual muscle groups. As you tense the following muscles, try to keep the rest of your muscles as relaxed as possible. Repeat each of the exercises three times:

1. Tighten your fists. Feel the tension radiating up your arms. Inhale deeply and hold the tension for several seconds. Exhale and let your hands relax.

2. Press your arms down against the ground or chair. Inhale and hold the tension for several seconds, concentrating on the sensation. Exhale and let your arms relax.

3. Shrug your shoulders up to your ears. Feel the tension in your neck and shoulders. Inhale and hold. Exhale and let your shoulders drop.

4. Frown and raise your eyebrows. Study the tightness in your face. Inhale and hold the tension. Then exhale and release.

5. Press your eyelids closed as tightly as possible. Inhale and hold. Exhale and open your eyes gently.

6. Open your mouth as wide as possible. Inhale and hold. Exhale and release your jaw.

7. Clench your jaw, biting your teeth down. Feel the tension spread across your skull. Inhale and hold. Exhale and release.

8. Inhale deeply into your belly, letting your chest expand. Hold the chest tension. Exhale and let your breath return to normal.

9. Tighten your abdominal muscles. Hold then relax.

10. Arch your back, chest up, and hips down. Inhale and hold. Exhale and release your back gently.

11. Tighten your hips and buttocks. Inhale and hold. Exhale and relax.

12. Tense your left leg, from thigh to heel. Inhale and hold. Exhale and relax.

13. Tense your right leg, from thigh to heel. Inhale and hold. Exhale and relax.

14. Curl your toes under. Inhale and hold. Exhale and relax.

15. Remaining still, scan your body. Experience the relaxation over your body. If you need to, return to areas of tension and repeat the exercise for that muscle group. Breathe naturally and deeply for several moments, experiencing the relaxed state. Gently and slowly, stand up.

66. Meditation (6)

Scientists continue to publish convincing data proving that meditation relieves pain, headaches, and makes you feel better. They are also showing that meditation changes the structure of your brain.

A rigorous <u>scientific study</u> was published in the journal *Biological Psychiatry*. It looked at the benefits of mindfulness meditation and how it changes people's brains and potentially improves overall health. The study was conducted at the Health and Human Performance Laboratory at Carnegie Mellon University.

The researchers recruited 35 unemployed men and women who were looking for work and were under significant stress. Half of the people were taught mindfulness meditation at a residential retreat center. The other half were provided sham mindfulness meditation, which involved relaxation and distraction from worries and stress.

All participants did stretching exercises, but the mindfulness group was asked to pay attention to bodily sensations, including unpleasant ones. The relaxation group was encouraged to talk to each other and ignore their bodily sensations.

After three days, all participants felt refreshed and better able to deal with the stress of unemployment. However, follow-up brain scans showed changes only in those who did mindfulness meditation. The scans showed more activity among the portions of their brains that process stress-related reactions and other areas related to focus and calm. By four months after the retreat, most people stopped meditating. However, the blood of those in the mindfulness meditation group still had much lower levels of interleukin-6, a marker of harmful inflammation, than the blood of those in the relaxation group.

These changes occurred after only 3 days of meditation. Long-term meditation practice produces stronger positive effects.

A study published in *The Journal of Neuroscience* compared the effect of meditation and placebo on pain. The study showed that mindfulness meditation provided greater pain relief than the placebo. Also, the brain scans could differentiate patterns of brain activity during meditation from those induced by a placebo pill.

The study involved seventy-five healthy, pain-free volunteers who were randomly assigned to one of four groups: mindfulness meditation, placebo meditation ("sham" meditation), placebo analgesic cream, or control.

Pain was induced by heat applied to the skin. The mindfulness meditation group reported that pain intensity was reduced by 27 percent and the emotional aspect of pain (how unpleasant it was) by 44 percent. In contrast, the placebo cream reduced the sensation of pain by 11 percent and the emotional aspect of pain by 13 percent.

Mindfulness meditation reduced pain by activating brain regions associated with the self-control of pain while the placebo cream lowered pain by reducing brain activity in pain-processing areas.

Another brain region, the thalamus, was deactivated during mindfulness meditation but was activated during all other conditions. This brain region serves as a gateway that determines if sensory information is allowed to reach higher brain centers. By deactivating this area, mindfulness meditation may have caused signals about pain to simply fade away, according to Dr. Zeidan, one of the researchers.

Mindfulness meditation was also significantly better at reducing pain intensity and pain unpleasantness than the placebo meditation. The placebo-meditation group had relatively small decreases in pain intensity (9%) and pain unpleasantness (24%). The study findings suggest that placebo meditation may have reduced pain through a relaxation effect that was associated with slower breathing.

This study is the first to show that mindfulness meditation does not relieve pain the way a placebo does. It also confirms previous observations that as little as four 20-minute daily sessions of mindfulness meditation could enhance pain treatment.

Another study has shown that an 8-week course of mindfulness meditation not only relieved pain but also made certain parts of the brain cortex measurably thicker.

Dr. Rebecca Wells and her colleagues published a study in the journal *Headache*, Meditation for Migraines: A Pilot Randomized Controlled Trial. It showed that mindfulness-based stress reduction, which is a form of meditation, "...had a beneficial effect on headache duration, disability, self-efficacy, and mindfulness."

There are several ways to learn meditation. You can listen to free podcasts by a wonderful psychologist Tara Brach. My favorite book to learn meditation by is *Mindfulness in Plain English* by B. Gunaratana. And of course, there is an app for that. Headspace.com and Calm.com are two of the more popular ones. You can also find local meditation courses offered by churches, community centers, and gyms.

Here is a simple guide to meditation (adapted from *The Headache Alternative: A Neurologist's Guide to Drug-Free Relief,* A. Mauskop and M. A. Brill, Dell 1997):

1. Find a comfortable position - lying down or sitting either on the floor or in a straight-backed chair. If sitting, keep your back straight, without being rigid, and let your hands rest in your lap.

2. Scan your body for tension from head to toe and relax your muscles. Unfurl your eyebrows and unclench your jaw. Release your shoulders, arms, and belly. Let your sitz bones sink into the chair or ground.

3. Be aware of the sensation of your body touching the floor (or firm surface).

4. Close your eyes if you feel like it's more comfortable.

5. Focus your mind on your breath as you inhale and exhale naturally. You can just focus on the sensation of air passing through your nostrils. Or, feel your belly going in and out with each breath.

6. Keep your mind focused on your breath.

7. When thoughts cross your mind, gently note them, let them pass, and return to your breathing. Each time this happens - and in the beginning, it will happen all the time - simply return to the breath. Almost everyone becomes frustrated and feels that this is a waste of time because the mind keeps wandering. But if you persevere, you will notice longer and longer periods without thinking.

8. Continue for 10 or 20 minutes. It's okay to set a timer.

9. Sit quietly for another minute.

You can use the breath as a focus, or select a word as a mantra. Any simple, positive word or name will do. Daily meditation is generally recommended to achieve the best results in health improvement. Try to practice once or twice a day, 10 or 20 minutes at a time. But it is better to sacrifice time for consistency; if you only have 5 minutes, do it. Just as long as you do it every day. Buddhists have a joke. You should meditate for 20 minutes every day. If you are too busy, you should meditate for an hour.

67. Praying and cursing (2)

Faith and prayer are the vitamins of the soul; man cannot live in health without them.

—Mahalia Jackson

Scientific studies on the effect of prayer are hard to do. Nevertheless, the power of prayer in a believer should not be underestimated. Some religious patients tell me that they do not need to meditate because they pray every day. I tell them that prayer is probably as effective as meditation if their prayer is not perfunctory, but devotional and they are not being distracted by other thoughts.

Migraines and meditation: does spirituality matter? This article in the *Journal of Behavioral Medicine* reported on a study that examined two questions. Is spiritual meditation more effective in enhancing pain tolerance and reducing migraine headache-related symptoms than secular meditation and relaxation? And does spiritual meditation create better mental, physical, and spiritual health outcomes than secular meditation and relaxation techniques? Eighty-three meditation-naïve people with frequent migraines were taught Spiritual Meditation, Internally Focused Secular Meditation, Externally Focused Secular Meditation, or Muscle Relaxation. The participants practiced these methods for 20 minutes a day for one month. The authors measured pain tolerance, headache frequency, and mental and spiritual health variables. Compared to the other three groups, people who practiced spiritual meditation had greater improvement in the frequency of migraine headaches, anxiety, and negative affect. They had greater increases in pain tolerance, headache-related self-efficacy, daily spiritual experiences, and existential well-being.

In an Iranian study <u>of 92 patients, the migraine prevention drug,</u> <u>propranolol, was significantly more effective when it was combined with prayer</u>. The prayer group participated in an 8-week, weekly, intercessory prayer program with each session lasting 45 minutes.

Cursing is the opposite of prayer. But it helps pain faster than prayer. Having given injections to thousands of patients, I know that some patients tolerate pain better if they curse during the procedure.

A British psychologist Richard Stephens seems to have made a career out of studying the effect of cursing on pain. His first paper *Swearing as a Response* *to Pain* appeared in 2009 in *NeuroReport.* It showed that swearing improves pain tolerance in volunteers whose hand was submerged in icy water.

His next paper published in 2011, *Swearing as a Response to Pain—Effect* *of Daily Swearing Frequency* was published in *The Journal of Pain.* In this study, Stephens looked at the effect of repeated daily swearing on experimental pain. The volunteers were again subjected to pain by submerging their hand into icy water. And the researchers again showed that swearing reduces pain. However, people who tended to swear frequently throughout the day had less of a pain-relieving effect than those who did not.

His 2020 article, *Swearing as a Response to Pain: Assessing Hypoalgesic* *Effects of Novel "Swear" Words,* was published in the *Frontiers in Psychology.* The authors show that made-up "swear" words are not as effective as the good old four-letter f-word.

The conclusion of this 6,500-word research paper suggests that there is still a lot more swearing ... I mean, studying to be done on this subject. Whether this is a good use of the British taxpayers' money is another matter. Perhaps the ultimate goal is to save the British National Health Service money by replacing pain medications with scientifically validated swear words.

68. Cognitive-behavioral therapy (7)

Life and death are in the power of the tongue.

—Proverbs 18:21.

Words are, of course, the most powerful drug used by mankind.

—Rudyard Kipling

Cognitive-behavioral therapy (CBT) has been proven to help the pain of headaches. Many people are skeptical about the value of psychological treatments. They often tell me to just get rid of their migraines and they will be fine. Unfortunately, sometimes it takes time to relieve chronic headaches and pain. So, while we are trying to find relief, it helps us to learn how to function better despite the pain. This involves learning how not to panic and become paralyzed by headaches, to inform and interact with family, friends, and employers who can be understanding and perhaps even helpful. Research indicates that people who take charge of their care, get involved in working with the doctor to find relief, learn relaxation techniques, rather than passively waiting for doctors to "fix" the problem, do better.

CBT, which usually involves relaxation training, is one way to improve your health. It usually involves 8 to 12 structured sessions. Here is an example of what might take place during these sessions:

1. Three-component CBT model (thoughts, feelings, behaviors), pain monitoring

2. Relaxation training (diaphragmatic breathing, progressive muscle relaxation, guided imagery)

3. Migraine trigger avoidance

4. Pain-fatigue cycle, activity pacing, and pleasant event scheduling

5. Identifying and challenging negative thoughts (Activity, Belief, Consequences, Dispute model)

6. Problem-solving skills training and assertive communication

7. Review and practice

8. Relapse prevention

Another form of CBT is Acceptance Commitment Therapy (ACT). When California researchers compared it to traditional CBT, <u>they found them to be equally effective in chronic pain patients</u>. However, those who received ACT reported a higher level of satisfaction. This is what a typical schedule of sessions of ACT looks like:

1. The limits of control (short and long-term costs and benefits; finger traps), focus on experience (body scan)

2. Values (what you care about, how you want to live your life)

3. Cognitive defusion (observing thoughts without trying to evaluate or change them)

4. Mindfulness (being in the moment, raisin exercise)

5. Committed action ("road map" connecting values, goals, actions, obstacles, and strategies)

6. Review and continued action in support of values

7. Moving forward

CBT is usually conducted by a social worker or a psychologist. Many people lack access to individual psychotherapy either owing to their location or to financial constraints. Group sessions are also effective. Online, web-based CBT is another good alternative. An Australian website ThisWayUp.org.au offers free CBT for anxiety, depression, chronic pain, and other problems. The psychologists who developed and run this site published results of their treatments in scientific journals. They showed that self-taught CBT can be effective. Here is a schedule of lessons for anxiety and depression on the ThisWayUp website:

Lesson 1: About anxiety and depression

Learn about your own symptoms of anxiety and/or depression, and learn to tackle the physical symptoms of anxiety/depression.

Lesson 2: Identifying thoughts and tackling low activity

Learn to identify the thought symptoms of anxiety/depression, and learn to tackle the behaviors associated with anxiety/depression.

Lesson 3: Tackling thoughts

Learn to tackle the thought symptoms of anxiety/depression.

Lesson 4: Tackling avoidance

Learn to tackle avoidance behaviors associated with anxiety/depression by facing your fears.

Lesson 5: Mastering your skills

Learn to master your ability to face your fears using graded exposure, and learn to cope with the distressing emotions associated with anxiety/depression.

Lesson 6: Staying well

Learn how to avoid relapses and how to keep getting better!

69. Psychotherapy (4)

Just as man cannot live without dreams, he cannot live without hope.

—Elie Wiesel

To live without hope is to cease to live.

—Fyodor Dostoyevsky

Dynamic, interpersonal, analytic, and other forms of psychotherapy are not forms of CBT but can be helpful for some people who suffer from chronic pain and migraines. This is not because chronic pain is due to a psychological problem, but because living with chronic pain is very difficult, often leading to feelings of brokenness and shame. Very often people's lifestyles are diminished as a result of chronic pain and migraine. Psychotherapy can help people adjust to these limitations, cope with the fear that a migraine will come on, and communicate to friends, family members, and colleagues about what they are suffering from in a way that does not exacerbate feelings of shame and self-blame. Although it is hard to quantify the efficacy of psychotherapy, it is clear that people with migraine and other forms of chronic pain can benefit from the emotional support that psychotherapy provides.

The largest study of short-term psychotherapy involved 228 chronic pain patients who received an average of 6 sessions delivered by 31 therapists. Psychiatric symptoms and interpersonal problems were assessed at three time points. Healthcare data from baseline year and three years following treatment came from independent governmental databases. The results indicated significant reductions in symptoms and interpersonal problems during treatment. The researchers also found successive reductions in yearly healthcare costs, reaching the normal population mean two years post-treatment. The authors concluded that "Within the limitations of the uncontrolled design, our study suggests that the intensive short-term dynamic psychotherapy may be both clinically effective and cost-effective for patients with chronic pain."

John Sarno, a prominent physiatrist, developed a treatment for low back pain which he described in his book, *Mind Over Back Pain*. Some of his ideas, like his belief that there is no correlation between chronic back pain and herniated discs, have been validated by research published in leading medical journals. He felt that anger, hurt, emotional pain, and sadness generated during your childhood or throughout your life is a major contributor to chronic pain, including migraines.

In the words of Oliver Sacks, "It now became apparent to me that many migraine attacks were drenched in emotional significance, and could not be usefully considered, let alone treated, unless their emotional antecedents and effects were exposed in detail.

Thus a rage-migraine may be regarded as a complex but stereotyped reaction to rage, in patients who experience this. ... The patient is stuffed, impacted, and bloated with anger. ... If migraines are put to a special use, they must have a particular meaning for the patient; they must stand for something; they must allude to something; they must represent something. Thus it will be possible for us to approach a migraine not only as a physical event, but as a peculiar form of symbolic drama into which the patient has translated important thoughts and feelings; if we do this we will then be faced with the task of interpreting it as we would interpret a dream, i.e. discovering the hidden meaning of the manifest symptoms."

Elie Wiesel, who became my patient in his 70s, spoke about his headaches at a conference that I organized in Israel in 2008. The full text of his lecture was published in the journal *Headache*. You can read it on my blog. Here is a brief excerpt:

"I got up this morning with a very, very bad headache. So, I said to my headache, "You won't win." I speak to my headache; I personalize it. I say, "I know who you are, and I know what you want, and it won't work." And the pain says to me, "Let's see, Wiesel." And so we fight.

Through my studies, I've discovered that many writers and artists and painters have suffered from headaches, and they have had their own distinctive methods of coping. Dumas used to place a wet cloth on his forehead. Hemingway used to do write standing, because this seemed to afford some relief. Many of the great writers had headaches. Perhaps writers have headaches because they are afraid of critics.

And to this day I have not found a way of handling my own headache except in my own fashion, which is to live with it. It hasn't slowed down my work. I teach full-time, and I am a very obsessive professor. In some 40 years, I don't think I've ever given the same course twice. I want to be the best student in the class. That's how I learn and grow with the students. And all that with my constant companion, this headache."

70. Hypnosis (3)

Hypnosis sounds like a magical solution to any health problem. It would be wonderful if you could be hypnotized out of your migraines. Although it is not a magical cure, hypnosis and self-hypnosis can help.

A study by Niamh Flynn of Galway, Ireland examined the effect of an online hypnosis program for the treatment of migraines. Forty-three participants were randomly assigned to a wait-list control or a treatment group. The treatment group received hypnosis recordings developed for the study. Pain catastrophizing, headache disability, migraine frequency, duration, severity, and medication usage were measured. There was a 48% reduction in the mean headache disability score in the treatment group and a 2% reduction in the control group. The mean pain catastrophizing score dropped by 60% in the treatment group. There was a significant between-group difference in the change in migraine duration but not frequency or severity.

Hypnosis was compared with propranolol and placebo in 28 children with migraines. Propranolol is a blood pressure medication proven to prevent migraines. Self-hypnosis reduced the frequency of migraine attacks much more than propranolol or placebo.

A scientific review of eighty-five studies of hypnosis for painful conditions, consisting of 3,632 participants established that hypnosis had pain-relieving effects for all pain outcomes. Some people are more susceptible to hypnosis than others and the efficacy was strongly influenced by hypnotic suggestibility and by the use of direct pain-relieving suggestions. Optimal pain relief was obtained when hypnosis included direct pain-relieving suggestions administered to those with high and medium suggestibility. Respectively, 42% and 29% had clinically meaningful reduction in pain. The authors concluded that hypnotic intervention can deliver meaningful pain relief for most people. Therefore, it may be an effective and safe alternative to pharmaceutical intervention.

DRUGS

Many drugs used for the treatment of migraines were originally developed for high blood pressure, epilepsy, or depression, and were later found to help migraines. Edward Liveing wrote in 1873: "...pharmaceutical remedies which are most serviceable in the treatment of megrim are the same which enjoy a reputation for the cure or relief of other maladies..." He also noted that "One circumstance common for the operation of pharmaceutical remedies... is the singular uncertainty of their curative influence." The drugs are different and much better now, but unfortunately, we still go by trial and error. This is true even for the newest "designer" drugs that are specifically developed to treat migraines.

The good news is that within the next twenty years, the exponential growth of computing power will enable us to do a quick and inexpensive analysis of your genetic makeup. This will predict your response to new and old treatments and we will thus no longer have to resort to trial and error to determine which medication is most likely to be helpful for you.

In the first decade of their use, all new drugs are very expensive. The reason for this is that it takes decades of research and billions of dollars to develop a new drug and to make sure that it is safe and effective. If companies are not allowed to recoup these costs and make a profit, private investment will dry up and innovation will slow down. Although governments could increase their support for drug research, it would be impossible to match the intense competitive atmosphere of biotechnology companies, which are funded by venture capital. Fortunately, all drugs eventually lose their patent protection and prices drop when the drug becomes "generic," making them much more affordable and more readily covered by insurance.

The first group of drugs that I will discuss is acute or abortive. They are taken as needed whenever a migraine strikes. The second group is preventive medications that are taken daily, whether or not migraine is occurring. Some drugs can be used for both purposes, and a few are listed under both categories.

To remind you, the numbers after each drug indicates my subjective overall grade on a scale of 1 to 10. This grade takes into account efficacy, safety, ease of use, and other factors.

Asterisk indicates that the drug or treatment is approved by the FDA or the European Medicines Agency.

Another disclaimer mentioned at the beginning of the book is that most of the scientific references do not imply that the treatment is scientifically proven. The reported improvement may be purely due to the placebo effect and other factors. This is also included in my overall grade.

Acute Treatments

All migraine drugs are more effective if taken early in the attack. Many people wait to see if a migraine will go away on its own, even if, in their prior experience, it never does. Often people will take an over-the-counter medicine before taking a prescription drug, even if that strategy rarely works. Some patients think that over-the-counter drugs are safer and are worried about taking a prescription drug. This is often not true.

Unfortunately, doctors do not prescribe triptans often enough even though they are the best drugs for severe migraines. In the US, doctors more often prescribe narcotic or opioid drugs while in Europe, non-steroidal anti-inflammatory drugs (NSAIDs). This results in less than optimal control of migraines. Poor control of individual migraine attacks can lead to an increase in their frequency. Some people go on to have migraines daily and these chronic migraines become more difficult to control.

The Israeli psychologist and economist, Nobel Prize winner Daniel Kahneman, wrote a fascinating book, *Thinking Fast and Slow*. In it, he suggests that there are easily correctable factors that may be contributing to poor decision making. The idea of mental energy is more than a mere metaphor, he said. Our nervous system consumes more glucose than most other parts of the body. Here is an excerpt from his book:

"A disturbing demonstration of depletion effect in judgment was reported in the *Proceedings of the National Academy of Sciences*. The unwitting participants in the study were eight parole judges in Israel. They spent entire days reviewing applications for parole. The cases were presented in random order, and the judges spent an average of 6 minutes on each case. Only 35% of requests are approved. The exact time of each decision was recorded *along with the times of the judges' three food breaks. The proportion of approved paroles spiked after each meal when about 65% of requests were granted. During the two hours until the judges' next meal, the approval rate drops to about zero just before the meal. The conclusion was that tired and hungry judges tend to fall back on the easier default position of denying requests for parole. Both fatigue and hunger probably play a role."*

A similar study was published in *JAMA Network Open* by the University of Minnesota researchers, providing hard data on the prescribing of opioid analgesics. The study evaluated 5,603 primary care practitioners who were involved in 678,319 primary care encounters for a painful condition.

Doctors were 33% more likely to prescribe an opioid pain medicine at the end of the workday than at the beginning. If the doctor was running an hour or more behind schedule he or she was 17% more likely to prescribe an opioid. The incidence of prescribing NSAIDs and referrals to physical therapy did not change.

For best results, you may want to try to see your doctor right after lunch and hope that he or she had time to eat. You may also want to eat before an important presentation, test, or another mentally demanding task.

Triptans

Sumatriptan, released in 1992, was the first drug specifically developed for the acute treatment of migraines. It is considered to be the gold standard in treating acute migraine. Sumatriptan and similar drugs have alleviated the suffering of millions of people. Unfortunately, almost three decades later millions of migraine sufferers still have not had access to these drugs.

Dr. Richard Lipton and his colleagues surveyed 15,133 migraine sufferers and found that only 37% had ever used a triptan and only 16% were using them at the time of the survey. Most patients took tablets, but 11% also tried either a nasal spray or an injection. Lack of efficacy (in 38%) and side effects (in 22%) were the most common reason for stopping the drug. The most common side effects were dizziness, nausea, and fatigue.

The lack of efficacy is often due to the suboptimal dose of a triptan that is prescribed. Many patients tell me that they've tried sumatriptan and it did not work. They've tried 25 or 50 mg. An effective dose for most patients is 100 mg. Most other triptans are available in two different strengths and the lower, less effective dose is often prescribed.

Another common problem is that patients who fail one triptan due to side effects or lack of efficacy are not prescribed a different triptan. Many of my patients find that one triptan is more effective than another or if one triptan causes side effects, a different one may not. Also, if a tablet does not work, an injection or a nasal spray might, especially in patients with a quick buildup of pain or when nausea is present. On the other hand, if two different triptans were tried on separate occasions and did not work at all, chances are that none of them will.

A big reason for the underutilization of triptans is the misdiagnosis of headaches. Almost half of the migraine sufferers are told that they have sinus or tension headaches, which means they are missing out on receiving effective treatment.

The safety of triptans is a concern of many physicians and patients. The package insert warns about strokes and heart attacks. If you have untreated hypertension, coronary artery disease, or many risk factors for coronary artery disease, you should not take triptans. However, the large majority of migraine sufferers are young women without these problems.

A panel of leading headache specialists published a "Consensus Statement: Cardiovascular Safety Profile of Triptans in the Acute Treatment of Migraine" that states, "The incidence of serious cardiovascular events with triptans in both clinical trials and clinical practice appears to be extremely low ".

In 2020, researchers at Kaiser Permanente in Southern California published a study of 189,684 patients with migraine, *Risk of Acute Myocardial Infarction, Heart Failure, and Death in Migraine Patients Treated with Triptans*. 130,656 of these patients were exposed to triptans. The authors concluded: "No association was found between exposure to triptans and an increased risk of cardiovascular events. These data provide reassurance regarding the cardiovascular safety of utilizing triptans for the medical management of migraine headaches."

You may still be able to take triptans if you have risk factors for coronary artery disease. But, you would need to have the condition of your coronary arteries checked regularly. This can be done with a coronary calcium scoring CT scan, stress test, or coronary angiogram.

According to the National Poison Data System, in five years (2014-2018), there were 328 overdoses with a triptan, none of which were fatal.

In most European countries triptans have been available without a prescription since 2007. This also attests to their safety.

80

A unique feature of rizatriptan is that the FDA-approved dose is up to three 10-mg tablets a day. It is also available in 5-mg tablets. All other triptans have a limit of only two of the highest available dose in one day. There is no significant difference between rizatriptan and most other triptans. Unfortunately, many doctors strictly adhere to the FDA guidelines, and these are just guidelines. They sternly warn patients not to exceed the FDA-recommended dose. The five most effective triptans (excluding naratriptan and frovatriptan) have a half-life of 2-3 hours, which means that half of a single dose is gone from your body in 2-3 hours. Naratriptan has a half-life of 6 hours and frovatriptan, 26 hours. Even if you were to take naratriptan three times a day it would not put you in any danger. Some of my patients know that one tablet of a triptan will not be enough for a severe attack and they take two at once. There is no evidence of any danger from doing that either. These dosages were arrived at by looking for an optimal dose that provides the best relief with the fewest side effects. For most people, the standard dose will work well, but some patients need higher amounts. In the case of eletriptan, we have 20 mg and 40 mg tablets in the US. In some European countries, it is available in 80 mg.

According to the FDA, you should not take two different triptans within 24 hours of each other. There is no good reason for such a prohibition. You are allowed to take a second dose of the same triptan two hours after the first dose. It makes no sense why, two hours later, you could not take a different one. There is no evidence of a negative interaction between different triptans. A <u>report in the journal Headache by Dr. John Rothrock and Veronica Morey describes 200 patients who "mixed triptans"</u> by taking a shot of sumatriptan two hours before or after a tablet of either rizatriptan, zolmitriptan, almotriptan, or eletriptan. He found that not only were there no problems, but patients were highly satisfied with this approach.

Sumatriptan was released in a pack of nine tablets. This was not because it is dangerous to take more, but because this was the average number of tablets people used in one month in clinical trials. Cost used to be another limiting factor, and some insurers still limit triptans to six or nine tablets a month. However, nine tablets of generic sumatriptan can now <u>be found for as little as $12,</u> so patients can bypass their insurance and buy additional tablets as long as doctors are willing to prescribe a higher amount.

Many doctors have another unfounded concern. They believe that frequent use of triptans will make migraines more frequent and severe, causing a medication overuse headache, or MOH. There is no good scientific evidence for this belief. It leads to thousands of headache sufferers being unfairly blamed for causing or worsening their headaches. This misconception causes many patients to be denied safe and effective treatment that could relieve their suffering and reduce disability. I have seen patients whose headaches worsen with frequent use of triptans and improve when triptans are stopped. The number of such patients is very small. For a great multitude of my patients, frequent use of triptans allows them to lead normal lives.

My <u>blog post on the daily use of triptans is by far the most popular I've written</u>, eliciting over 300 comments. Many patients comment on how relieved they are to know that they are not risking their lives by taking triptans often or even daily. Many express their frustration about not being able to find a doctor who would prescribe a sufficient amount of this life-changing medicine.

Here are a few of these poignant comments:

"I had been taking triptans for over 20 years up to 20 times per month. They have been a miracle for me."

"I have been on daily sumatriptan for 4 years and after 30 years of suffering with chronic migraines, these have been the best 4 years of my life! Out of the blue, my regular physician decided I should see a headache specialist and now neither of them will prescribe more than 6 pills a month."

"OMG, I am so happy that I found your blog. If I listen to my body, it tells me the same that you do about triptans and other drugs used for migraine. I tolerate triptans very well and take them almost daily, even though I have managed to decrease the number since I reached menopause."

"I take sumatriptan an average of 12-15 times a month and without it, I wouldn't be able to function. I know it doesn't cause MOH for me, because I sometimes have been able to go without it for 7-11 days. Anytime I tried to delay taking it, it only makes the migraine worse and won't stop until I take it."

"I've done the botox, depakote, and countless other preventatives. I'm 57 and have been fighting this since I was 18. I am otherwise healthy, good weight, etc. I'm currently a surreptitious daily triptan user – as my Doctor is putting her foot down at about 18 a month."

"I'm almost 80 and have suffered from migraines on and off since I was a teenager. My triggers are barometric pressure and stress. Like others on this forum, I've tried every therapy, preventative and medication, including botox, over the years and the ONLY thing that works for me are triptans. In the past few years my migraines have become chronic and Amerge has been my lifesaver. My family doctor retired this year and the new young doctor who took over her practice will not prescribe Amerge for me, citing my age and risk of stroke. This despite the fact I have annual stress tests and my heart is in great shape. I am also otherwise very healthy and active. The last thing I want is to spend the rest of my senior years lying, nauseous, in a dark room. The doctor wants me to handle these vicious headaches with Tylenol, which is like trying to kill an elephant with a fly swatter. Do you have any other suggestions?"

"I have daily migraines, and have been taking triptans daily for several years. Yesterday, my neurologist, after hearing I was under increased stress because my husband just lost his job, decided that I should be limited to 15 triptans a month, and to deal with the rest via biofeedback and "mind over matter." She claimed that triptans cause stroke and cardiac problems."

A small minority of leading headache specialists feel that MOH due to triptans is a myth. Drs. Ann Scher of Uniformed Services University, Paul Rizzoli and Elizabeth Loder, both of Brigham and Women's Hospital published an article in a leading neurology journal, *Neurology*, entitled, *Medication overuse headache. An entrenched idea in need of scrutiny*. The abstract of this article reads:

"It is a widely accepted idea that medications taken to relieve acute headache pain can paradoxically worsen headache if used too often. This type of secondary headache is referred to as medication overuse headache (MOH); previously used terms include rebound headache and drug-induced headache. In the absence of consensus about the duration of use, amount, and type of medication needed to cause MOH, the default position is conservative. A common recommendation is to limit treatment to no more than 10 or 15 days per month (depending on medication type) to prevent headache frequency progression. Medication withdrawal is often recommended as a first step in the treatment of patients with frequent headaches. Existing evidence, however, does not provide a strong basis for such causal claims about the relationship between medication use and frequent headache. Observational studies linking treatment patterns with headache frequency are by their nature confounded by indication. Medication withdrawal studies have mostly been uncontrolled and often have high dropout rates. Evaluation of this evidence suggests that only a minority of patients required to limit the use of symptomatic medication may benefit from treatment limitation. Similarly, only a minority of patients deemed to be overusing medications may benefit from withdrawal. These findings raise serious questions about the value of withholding or withdrawing symptom-relieving medications from people with frequent headaches solely to prevent or treat MOH. The benefits of doing so are smaller, and the harms larger, than currently recognized. The concept of MOH should be viewed with more skepticism. Until the evidence is better, we should avoid dogmatism about the use of symptomatic medication. Frequent use of symptom-relieving headache medications should be viewed more neutrally, as an indicator of poorly controlled headaches, and not invariably a cause."

71. Sumatriptan*, tablets (7), nasal (6), injection (9), with naproxen (8)

Sumatriptan (Imitrex, Imigran) remains the most popular triptan. It lost patent protection years ago and many manufacturers make generic copies, thus dramatically reducing its price. Sumatriptan is available in combination with naproxen (Treximet). This combination is more effective than either drug alone but remains expensive.

Sumatriptan is available in 25, 50, and 100 mg strength. The starting dose for most patients is 100 mg. If after two hours one tablet has not relieved your migraine, take another 100 mg tablet.

The sumatriptan nasal spray does not work as well as the tablets but the newer nasal forms of sumatriptan (Onzetra, Tosymra) work better. However, they are much more expensive. Some patients complain of an unpleasant taste from the sumatriptan spray. This problem can be avoided by sucking on hard candy while taking the spray. This will carry the saliva out of the mouth down the throat and the drug will not reach the mouth. Others find nasal spray irritating and prefer an injection.

The sumatriptan injection is the most effective treatment for acute migraine. <u>Over 80% of patients respond</u> to it. Unfortunately, the injections are highly underutilized. The doctors are not familiar with them, forget to offer them, and are afraid to prescribe them. The misperception is that the side effects are common. Or they incorrectly assume that patients will not be receptive to the idea of injecting themselves.

The injection begins to work within 10-15 minutes. It can quickly restore one to normal functioning. The injections are particularly useful when tablets do not work well or fast enough. The ideal candidates for injections are people who wake up with a severe migraine, have a rapid onset of intense pain, or have pronounced nausea or vomiting with their attacks.

Tightness in the jaw, neck, or chest is more common with the injection than with the tablet. This sensation can be frightening but it is not dangerous and is not related to the heart. It usually subsides in about 15 minutes.

The injection is available in a vial and an easy-to-use autoinjector. Each shot contains 3 mg, 4 mg, or 6 mg of sumatriptan. The most commonly used dose is 6 mg. If cost is an issue, a vial is significantly cheaper than an autoinjector. With the vial, you will also need a separate prescription for syringes.

72. Rizatriptan* (7)

Rizatriptan (Maxalt, Maxalt MLT) is one of the two triptans available in an orally disintegrating tablet that melts in your mouth. The tablet melts in your mouth and does not require water to take it. This is important for those who are so nauseated that they cannot drink even a small amount of fluid without throwing up. It also means that you can take it when water is not available. We know that the earlier you take an abortive drug the better the results. Rizatriptan comes in 5 and 10 mg tablets. You can take one tablet and if the pain is not completely gone, take a second tablet two hours later. The maximum daily dose is 30 mg.

Rizatriptan is approved for children as young as 6. For young children, 5 mg is the starting dose but the FDA does not offer guidance as to the maximum daily dose for children. Just like with adults, taking 5 mg up to three times a day is safe.

73. Zolmitriptan* (7)

Zolmitriptan (Zomig, Zomig ZMT, Zomig NS) is available in tablets, orally disintegrating tablets, and nasal spray. The nasal spray is approved for children 12 and older. Both tablets and the spray are available in 2.5 mg and 5 mg strength.

The advantage of the nasal spray is that it tends to have a faster onset of action and it can be taken when severe nausea or vomiting precludes the use of oral medications. My impression is that zolmitriptan spray is more effective than sumatriptan spray. The amount of fluid in a single dose of Zomig is less than that in Imitrex and the spray droplets are of smaller size, leading to better retention of fluid in the nasal passages and to better absorption.

Zolmitriptan nasal spray is expensive because it is still available only as a branded product. It will lose its patent protection in 2021.

74. Eletriptan*(7)

Eletriptan (Relpax, Relert) is similar to the other five fast-acting triptans. For some people, eletriptan is more effective than other triptans. This is my subjective impression and it is not supported by any scientific study.

Eletriptan is available in 20 and 40 mg tablets with the maximum FDA-approved daily dose of 80 mg. In some European countries, eletriptan is sold in 80 mg tablets and the maximum approved daily dose is 160 mg.

75. Almotriptan*(7)

Almotriptan (Axert, Almogran) is another fast-acting triptan. It is approved for adults and children as young as 12. The drug is available in 6.25 mg and 12.5 mg strength. The maximum daily dose is 25 mg. Almotriptan is not as widely used because it was the sixth triptan to be approved by the FDA.

76. Naratriptan* (6)

Naratriptan (Amerge, Naramig) has a longer half-life of 6 hours. This results in a longer duration of action. The duration of the effect is not important for most migraine sufferers. A short-lasting but quick-acting drug can stop the migraine process and there is no need for it to linger in the body. In some patients, however, sumatriptan or another short-acting triptan may relieve symptoms for 4-6 hours, and then the migraine returns. Taking a second dose often works, but not always. Those patients can benefit from taking naratriptan. Many patients find naratriptan to be milder in terms of side effects compared to other triptans.

The longer half-life makes naratriptan better suited for mini-prophylaxis – taking a drug daily for several days to prevent a predictable menstrual migraine. Sumatriptan and frovatriptan have also been shown to work for mini-prophylaxis.

77. Frovatriptan* (5)

Frovatriptan (Frova) is probably the least effective triptan. This is in part because it takes the longest to start working. On the positive side, its half-life is 26 hours. This means that the body clears out half of it within 26 hours.

When the speed of onset is not crucial, which is when migraine develops slowly over a few hours, frovatriptan has the advantage of a longer effect. However, if it does not provide good relief to begin with, the amount of time it stays in the body is irrelevant. Short-acting triptans work quickly and stop the migraine attack.

Frovatriptan is sometimes used for "mini-prophylaxis" of menstrual migraines – it is taken the day before the expected menstrual migraine and throughout the period.

Unlike other triptans, frovatriptan is available only in one strength – 2.5 mg. You can take up to 2 tablets a day, at least 2 hours apart.

NSAIDs

NSAIDs are effective pain medications. They reduce inflammation that occurs during a migraine attack. Millions of people take these drugs for various forms of arthritis and almost every type of pain. Occasional use of these drugs carries little risk. The risk increases with higher doses and prolonged use.

All NSAIDs except for aspirin carry a warning about possible heart complications. This is of no concern for the majority of migraine sufferers who tend to be young healthy women. Even in older patients with a few risk factors for heart disease, infrequent use of an NSAID is not going to cause a heart attack.

However, even occasional use of NSAIDs can cause gastrointestinal (GI) side effects – a stomach ulcer or heartburn (gastroesophageal reflux disease – GERD). All NSAIDs can cause bleeding ulcers which can be life-threatening. If you take an NSAID infrequently and do not have stomach problems such as reflux or ulcers, take it on an empty stomach. This will make the drug absorb and work faster.

All NSAIDs, which are so-called blood thinners, can cause increased bleeding and bruising. Prolonged use of large amounts of NSAIDs can damage kidneys <u>and cause tinnitus (ringing in the ears) and hearing loss</u>.

Frequent intake of NSAIDs is thought to lead to medication overuse headache. This happens very infrequently and the entire concept of MOH remains controversial (see the chapter on triptans above). Frequent or daily intake of NSAIDs is not the best way to manage frequent migraines. Many preventive therapies may be more effective and safer.

78. Diclofenac*(6)

Diclofenac (Voltaren) is available as a 50 mg tablet. Powdered diclofenac (Cambia), is specifically approved by the FDA for the treatment of migraine headaches. It works faster because the powder gets dissolved in a glass of water and the liquid solution tends to be absorbed faster than a solid pill. Cambia has a licorice taste, so if you are born disliking licorice – yes, it is an inherited trait – this drug is not for you.

The powdered form is expensive and the insurers rightfully want you to first try the same dose of 50 mg of the inexpensive generic diclofenac in a tablet form. Drinking a full glass of water will speed up the dissolution of the tablet and in some patients could potentially match the efficacy of Cambia.

79. Naproxen (6)

Naproxen (Naprosyn) and naproxen sodium (Aleve, Anaprox) are popular over-the-counter (OTC) and prescription drugs. They are often used for the treatment of migraine headaches. Naproxen sodium absorbs and works faster than naproxen.

A combination of 500 mg of naproxen sodium with 85 mg of sumatriptan (Treximet) is approved by the FDA for the treatment of acute migraine attacks.

Naproxen sodium alone, while not specifically approved for the treatment of migraines, is widely considered to be an effective drug. A review of several double-blind studies confirmed this fact. Naproxen and naproxen sodium have the advantage of providing a longer duration of effect than ibuprofen or aspirin.

OTC naproxen sodium (Aleve) is available in 220 mg tablets, gelcaps, and liquid gels. Liquid gels tend to work faster. The maximum recommended dose is 660 mg a day. Prescription naproxen is sold in 500 mg tablets and naproxen sodium in 550 mg ones. The maximum daily dose for naproxen by prescription is 1,500 mg and for naproxen sodium, 1,100 mg.

80. Meloxicam (5)

Meloxicam (Mobic) is a non-steroidal anti-inflammatory drug (NSAID) that is approved for the treatment of rheumatoid arthritis and osteoarthritis in adults and juvenile rheumatoid arthritis in children older than 2 years. Meloxicam tends to have fewer gastrointestinal side effects than some other NSAIDs, according to a large international study.

Although there have not been any trials of meloxicam for the acute or prophylactic treatment of migraine headaches, it is probably as effective as other NSAIDs that have been tested for migraines. One advantage of meloxicam is that the effect of a single dose lasts all day. This makes it particularly suitable for the prevention of migraine attacks. It is also available in liquid form, which works faster than a solid tablet. The speed of onset is important when using it for acute therapy – faster-acting drugs tend to be more effective.

Meloxicam tablets are available in 7.5 and 15 mg strength. The maximum daily dose is 15 mg.

81. Indomethacin (5)

Indomethacin (Indocin, Indocid) is one of the oldest and strongest NSAIDs, but it is rarely used for the treatment of migraines. It has a higher chance of causing GI side effects than other NSAIDs, but some patients tolerate it well, especially if it is used infrequently. In addition to capsules, indomethacin is available as a rectal suppository. Rectal administration reduces but does not eliminate GI side effects and provides faster onset of effect than an oral capsule. Even if nausea is not present, migraine is often accompanied by gastric stasis. This means that the absorption of oral drugs is slowed down. Rectal suppositories are less popular in the US than they are in Europe. The dose of oral indomethacin is 25, 50, or 75 mg taken up to three times a day. It is also available in a long-acting tablet. Suppositories contain 50 mg. The maximum daily dose is 150 mg.

Indomethacin has some unique properties that differentiate it from other NSAIDs. It is often the only NSAID that is effective for episodic and chronic paroxysmal hemicrania and hemicrania continua. The dose of indomethacin needed to control these types of headaches sometimes goes up to 225 mg a day. These headaches are often mistaken for migraines and are described at the end of this book.

82. Celecoxib (5)

Celecoxib (Celebrex) is an NSAID that belongs to a subclass of selective COX-2 inhibitors. COX-2 inhibitors tend to have fewer GI side effects compared to other NSAIDs. It is available in 50, 100, 200, and 400 mg strength. The maximum daily dose is 400 mg.

400 mg of Celecoxib was shown by Singaporean doctors to be as effective as 550 mg of naproxen for the acute treatment of migraine headaches.

A new formulation of 120 mg of celecoxib solution (Elyxyb) was recently approved by the FDA specifically for the acute treatment of migraines.

83. Mefenamic acid* (5)

Mefenamic acid (Ponstel, Ponstan) is similar to other NSAIDs and is effective for acute migraine attacks.

Mefenamic acid is popular for the treatment of menstrual migraines. This is probably because it is approved to not only treat mild or moderate pain, but also dysmenorrhea, or pain of menstruation. In a small study conducted by a doctor from Dubai, mefenamic acid was found to be specifically effective for the treatment of menstrual migraines, which can be more severe and more difficult to treat than non-menstrual attacks.

Mefenamic acid was found to be superior to acetaminophen by Dr. Jes Olesen and his colleagues in Denmark. This is no surprise since acetaminophen has little antiinflammatory action and therefore does not reduce inflammation that occurs during a migraine attack.

According to a study by Finnish doctors, mefenamic acid was as effective as ergotamine, but ergotamine caused more side effects, especially nausea. Ergotamine was the mainstay of migraine treatment before the introduction of triptans in 1992.

For the treatment of pain and primary dysmenorrhea, the initial dose is 500 mg, followed by 250 mg every 6 hours, as needed.

84. Ketorolac injection (7)

Ketorolac (Toradol) is available in a tablet and injection. In a tablet form, it is no more effective than ibuprofen, naproxen, or any other NSAID, but has more side effects and its use is limited to 5 days. Ketorolac as an injection, however, is a unique and useful drug. It provides pain relief comparable to that of opioid (narcotic) drugs without the side effects or addiction potential of those drugs.

Intravenous ketorolac has been proven to be very effective for the treatment of severe migraine attacks. A study performed by Dr. Benjamin Friedman and his colleagues at the emergency department of the Montefiore Medical Center in the Bronx compared intravenous infusion of 30 mg of ketorolac with an infusion of 10 mg of metoclopramide (Reglan) and 1,000 mg of valproate (Depacon). There were over 100 patients in each group, making this a highly reliable study. Ketorolac and metoclopramide were more effective than valproate, but metoclopramide caused severe restlessness in 6 (6%) of patients.

Doctors from the University of Texas compared <u>an intramuscular injection of 60 mg of ketorolac to an intravenous infusion of 25 mg of chlorpromazine (Thorazine) and found them to be equally effective</u>. Both prochlorperazine and chlorpromazine carry a risk of restlessness, involuntary movements, and sedation.

A review of eight published trials of ketorolac found it to be more effective than meperidine (Demerol) and sumatriptan and a little less effective than metoclopramide, chlorpromazine, and prochlorperazine. However, ketorolac lacks the addiction potential and the risk of severe restlessness, sedation, and involuntary movements.

We give intravenous ketorolac to our patients whose migraine has not responded to an oral triptan, an infusion of magnesium, or injection of sumatriptan. An intravenous dose of 60 mg is no more effective than 30 mg. Even 15 mg can provide good relief. We usually give 30 mg. The maximum daily dose by injection or infusion is 120 mg.

85. Aspirin (6)

<u>Aspirin is a very effective migraine drug</u>. A <u>rigorous analysis of three studies showed that 1,000 mg of effervescent aspirin is as effective as 50 mg of sumatriptan while causing fewer side effects</u>.

Aspirin has several features that distinguish it from other NSAIDs. While other NSAIDs can cause heart problems, aspirin is widely used to prevent them. It is also very effective for the prevention of different types of cancer.

It has a stronger and longer-lasting anti-clumping effect on platelets. This is probably why some patients find aspirin to be more effective than any other NSAID.

For a faster onset of action <u>and less stomach irritation</u>, I recommend an effervescent form of aspirin which also contains an antacid, sodium bicarbonate (Alka Seltzer). In Europe, effervescent forms of medications are much more popular than in the US and a 343-patient <u>study of an effervescent form of 1,000 mg of aspirin found it to be highly effective for the treatment of acute migraines</u>.

86. Ibuprofen* (6)

Ibuprofen (Advil, Motrin, Nuprin, Nurofen) is very effective for migraine headaches. It is available with and without a prescription and is specifically approved by the FDA for the treatment of migraines. This means that it has been studied in large placebo-controlled trials to prove that it is safe and effective. Ibuprofen was shown to be more effective than acetaminophen in children.

OTC ibuprofen is sold in 200 mg strength. The adult dose is 400 mg, while in children the dose is 10 mg per kilogram of weight. The maximum daily dose of OTC ibuprofen is 1,200 mg. Ibuprofen by prescription is available in 400, 600, and 800 mg strength with the maximum daily dose of 3,200 mg. I would not recommend taking the maximum dose because of potential side effects. It is better to try a different NSAID or a different drug that may work better and with a lower chance of side effects.

A liquified form of ibuprofen (Advil Liquigels, Advil Migraine) and liquid ibuprofen for children tend to work faster than a solid tablet.

87. Aspirin/caffeine/acetaminophen* (6)

A combination of aspirin, acetaminophen, and caffeine (Excedrin Migraine, Anadin Extra, Goody's Powder) is popular in many countries. It is approved by the FDA for the treatment of migraines and is available without a prescription. The studies that led to the FDA approval showed that each ingredient contributed to the efficacy of the combination. It works well for many people, which explains its popularity.

Each tablet usually contains 65 mg of caffeine. The role of caffeine in treating headaches is described below. The problem is that caffeine is proven to cause medication overuse headache (MOH).

Other side effects are related to aspirin – with frequent use it can cause upset stomach, ulcers, and bruising.

Gepants

Gepants work by blocking the same calcitonin gene-related peptide (CGRP) pathway as the injectable monoclonal antibodies (mAbs) that are used for the prevention of migraine attacks. mAbs include erenumab, fremanezumab, galcanezumab, and eptinezumab and are described in the section on preventive drugs.

The average cost of developing a new drug is $2.6 billion, making new drugs very expensive. This means that insurance companies will require that migraine patients first try and fail generic versions of a triptan, such as sumatriptan (Imitrex), or have a contraindication to taking a triptan. Contraindications for the use of triptans include cardiovascular disease (coronary artery disease, strokes, heart attacks, etc.), uncontrolled hypertension, and a few other conditions. Gepants appear to be safe in such patients and have a low incidence of side effects.

Oral triptans work well in about 50-60% of patients, which leaves millions of migraine sufferers without effective abortive therapy. For these patients, the introduction of gepants can be life-changing.

88. Ubrogepant* (7)

Ubrogepant (Ubrelvy) is the first oral anti-CGRP drug to be approved by the FDA for the acute treatment of migraine attacks with and without aura. So far, it is only approved for adults.

The recommended dose is 50 mg or 100 mg and it is best taken at the onset of a migraine. If needed, a second 50 mg or 100 mg tablet can be taken at least 2 hours after the initial dose. The maximum amount for 24 hours is 200 mg. Ubrogepant can be taken with or without food.

The side effects are mild and infrequent. The most common one is nausea, seen in 2% of those receiving placebo, 2% of those on 50 mg of ubrogepant, and 3% of patients taking 100 mg. The second most common side effect is sleepiness, present in 1% of patients taking placebo, 2% of those taking 50 mg, and 3% taking 100 mg.

89. Rimegepant* (7)

Rimegepant (Nurtec ODT) is the second gepant to be approved for the acute treatment of migraine headaches with and without aura. It is also approved only for adults.

Since there have been no head-to-head trials comparing the two gepants, it is hard to say if one is better than the other. According to clinical trials, they are very similar. This does not mean that they will be equally effective or cause the same side effects in a particular patient. As with triptans and other drugs, some patients strongly prefer one over another.

One difference is that rimegepant is an orally disintegrating tablet and does not require water, while ubrogepant is a solid tablet that is taken with water. This makes rimegepant easier to take on the go and could be easier to take for patients with severe nausea. Another minor difference is that the dose of rimegepant is 75 mg that is taken only once a day. This can be both an advantage and a disadvantage. The instructions are simple: take one tablet once on the day you have a migraine. Ubrogepant can be taken a second time, which adds to its overall efficacy.

The most common side effect of rimegepant is also nausea which occurred in 2% of patients compared with 0.4% of those on placebo.

Ditans

90. Lasmiditan*(4)

Lasmiditan (Reyvow) is the first (and probably the last) drug in the class of ditans. Like the triptans, it works through the serotonin system. However, it activates 5-HT_{1F} serotonin receptors, while triptans activate 5-HT_{1B} and 5-HT_{1D} receptors. This confers an advantage in that lasmiditan does not cause constriction of coronary arteries, which can happen with triptans. Therefore, patients with a history of a heart attack, angina, or multiple risk factors for vascular disease who cannot take triptans, now have another safe option in addition to gepants.

Lasmiditan may also be effective in patients for whom triptans and gepants are ineffective, partially effective, or cause side effects.

Lasmiditan is available in 50 mg and 100 mg tablets and the recommended dose is 50, 100, or 200 mg taken once a day.

Side effects are generally mild to moderate and the most frequent ones include dizziness, fatigue, tingling, drowsiness, nausea, and muscle weakness. Two driving studies showed that lasmiditan may cause significant driving impairment. Do not drive for 8 hours after taking this medicine.

Lasmiditan is a non-narcotic medication but is a controlled drug with low abuse potential and no evidence of physical dependence.

Other drugs

91. Acetaminophen (4)

Many migraine sufferers do not find acetaminophen (Tylenol, Panadol), known in Europe as paracetamol, to be strong enough to treat migraine headaches. It is not approved by the FDA to treat migraines. Nevertheless, it is one of the most popular drugs for all kinds of pain, including migraines. Double-blind placebo-controlled trials have proven that acetaminophen does relieve pain and associated symptoms of migraine headaches.

One such study published by Dr. Richard Lipton and his colleagues compared 1,000 mg of acetaminophen with a placebo in 351 migraine sufferers. After 2 hours, 58% in the acetaminophen group and 39% in the placebo group reported relief. Twice as many had no pain at all after 2 hours in the acetaminophen group compared to placebo – 22% vs 11%. No side effects were reported in either group. This study excluded patients with very severe attacks – those who needed to lie down and those who had vomiting more than 20% of the time.

Acetaminophen can help some patients with milder migraines and can be a useful adjunct to a prescription drug, such as sumatriptan, especially if ibuprofen, naproxen, and other NSAIDs are contraindicated or cause upset stomach or other side effects. Acetaminophen has fewer side effects than NSAIDs. It should not be used at high doses for months or years because it can cause liver damage. Liver damage can even occur from a shorter exposure to acetaminophen if it is regularly combined with alcohol.

Acetaminophen usually comes in 325 mg and 500 mg strength. The maximum single dose is 1,000 mg. It can be taken every 6 hours for a total of not more than 3,000 mg. Some people try taking more than 1,000 mg at once. This is futile since acetaminophen has a ceiling effect. This means that you cannot get more relief by increasing the dose beyond 1,000 mg. All you get is more side effects.

92. Dexamethasone (4)

Dexamethasone (Decadron) is a strong corticosteroid or steroid anti-inflammatory medication. It is similar to prednisone, methylprednisolone, and other steroids. Because inflammation is part of the migraine process and because NSAIDs work well for migraines, you'd expect that steroids would also be effective. And they do help. In a blinded study, 4 mg of dexamethasone given along with 10 mg of rizatriptan was more effective than rizatriptan alone and it reduced the rate of migraine recurrence. When dexamethasone is given intravenously in an emergency room setting it reduces the rate of migraine recurrence.

The usual oral and intravenous dose of dexamethasone is between 4 mg and 12 mg. Steroids have a multitude of potential side effects. These include anxiety, feeling "hyper", depression, insomnia, dizziness, upset stomach, increased blood sugar, among others. This is why steroids should not be used unless several other types of drugs have failed to stop an attack.

Some doctors prefer a 6-day tapering course of methylprednisolone (Medrol pack). The first-day dose in this regimen is 24 mg. It is equivalent to 4.5 mg of dexamethasone. In my experience, it is probably more effective to start with a stronger dose of a steroid drug and give it for a shorter time.

Steroids have a multitude of potential side effects. These include anxiety, or feeling "hyper", depression, insomnia, dizziness, upset stomach, increased blood sugar, and many others. This is why steroids should not be used unless several other types of drugs failed to stop an attack.

93. Caffeine (4)

Three hundred and fifty years ago, a British doctor, Thomas Willis who is regarded as the father of neurology, wrote that drinking strong coffee is the only medicine worth recommending to all migraine patients. Edward Liveing also advocated the use of caffeine for migraines in his 1873 classic text, *On Megrim, Sick-Headache.*

An intravenous infusion of 60 mg of caffeine citrate for an acute migraine showed significant relief within an hour of infusion. This study was published in 2015 in the *Journal of Caffeine Research* (yes, such a journal exists).

Caffeine is not a strong pain killer and is mostly used as an adjunct to other medications. It is combined with NSAIDs, acetaminophen, and prescription drugs such as butalbital.

Besides coffee, tea, and energy drinks, you can buy caffeine tablets in a pharmacy. Caffeine tablets usually contain 100 or 200 mg of caffeine. A dose of up to 400 mg a day is considered safe. The largest cup of coffee you can buy at Starbucks – Venti – contains 415 mg of caffeine.

Excessive intake of caffeine in medications or diet can cause restlessness and shakiness, insomnia, dizziness, rapid or abnormal heart rhythm, dehydration, anxiety, and physical dependency. It can also worsen your headaches. (See section 16).

94. Butalbital (2)

Butalbital, a short-acting barbiturate, is one of the three ingredients in headache drugs such as Fioricet, Fiorinal, Esgic, and their generic equivalents. Fiorinal and Fioricet derive their name from the Montefiore Headache Clinic, where they were developed over 60 years ago. In those days, extensive clinical trials were not required by the FDA and drugs were approved without much testing. These drugs are approved only for the treatment of tension-type headaches. They have never been shown to be effective for migraines, although this is what they are mostly used for. Fioricet and Esgic contain butalbital, caffeine, and acetaminophen. In Fiorinal acetaminophen is replaced with aspirin.

Neurologists have a strong aversion to this drug. General practitioners and obstetricians tend to like it because these are very old drugs and they are very familiar with them. The reasons neurologists dislike them are the addictive potential of butalbital and the worsening of headaches from caffeine. I've seen patients who admitted that they often take Fioricet to relieve anxiety. Some of them become physically dependent and addicted to it. My most memorable patient was one who took 20 to 30 tablets every day. I had to admit her to the hospital for detoxification. In patients who take more than 5-6 tablets a day sudden discontinuation can lead to an epileptic seizure. Withdrawal from caffeine worsens headaches, for which sumatriptan tablets or injections can help. Botox injections and other preventive migraine drugs can also make the withdrawal process less painful.

I must admit that I do have a very small number of patients whose migraines respond well to butalbital-containing drugs. They either did not respond or had contraindications to NSAIDs and triptans. Also, they do not show any signs of tolerance – that is, needing to take ever-increasing amounts of these drugs.

95. Ergotamine* (5)

Ergotamine was introduced over 70 years ago and for decades was the best migraine medicine. It was introduced when rigorous clinical trials were not required for the launch of a drug and <u>the evidence for its efficacy is modest</u>.

One milligram of ergotamine is often combined with 100 mg of caffeine (Cafergot) but it is also available as a 2-mg tablet that dissolves under the tongue and as a rectal suppository. Its main side effect is nausea which can be addressed by taking it with metoclopramide or another nausea medication. Just like triptans, it is contraindicated in people with circulation problems –

coronary, cerebral, or peripheral vascular disease. The maximum weekly dose of ergotamine is 10 mg.

Ergotamine is rarely used because it can cause severe nausea and because NSAIDs and triptans can be more effective.

96. Dihydroergotamine injection* (8), nasal*(4)

Intravenous dihydroergotamine (DHE-45) is one of the most effective migraine medications. It was introduced in 1943 and has been the go-to drug for migraines that do not respond to other medications. I consider using dihydroergotamine (DHE) after the failure of oral triptans, NSAIDs, steroid drugs, injections of ketorolac, sumatriptan, and metoclopramide, and sometimes, nerve blocks. Nausea and vomiting are common side effects, which is why I give it only if other drugs fail.

The Raskin protocol, named after Neil Raskin who was a headache specialist in San Francisco, consists of giving IV DHE with metoclopramide every 8 hours for several days to break a persistent migraine attack that does not respond to other measures. The Raskin protocol is typically administered in a hospital. Sometimes, however, a modified version can be used in the office. One infusion is given in the morning and the second one in the late afternoon. I usually pretreat patients with ondansetron or metoclopramide to prevent severe nausea and vomiting from DHE. Some patients don't have nausea with their migraines and may not need to get nausea medication beforehand.

Some of my patients give themselves a shot of DHE under the skin, subcutaneously at home. Subcutaneous injection is not as effective as an intravenous infusion. But for some patients, it works well and they can avoid coming to the clinic. Some take an oral nausea medication or even self-inject a nausea drug before giving themselves an injection of DHE.

DHE nasal spray (Migranal) has been available for over a decade. Its approval was based on a double-blind trial in 348 patients. The results of this trial are impressive, but in clinical practice, I do not find it to be as effective as the study suggests.

Two companies are developing a powdered form of DHE for intranasal delivery and the preliminary data suggests a much better efficacy than the nasal spray.

97. Propofol (3)

Propofol (Diprivan) was originally developed for general anesthesia during surgery. Smaller amounts were found to work well for "conscious sedation" to induce a semiconscious state for minor procedures such as colonoscopies.

In small doses, propofol appears to be effective for the treatment of migraines. A 2019 review of nine studies and case reports showed that "Propofol may be an effective rescue therapy for patients presenting to the ED for acute migraine, but its place in therapy based on the limited available evidence is unknown." ED stands for emergency department.

Propofol was also tested for the emergency room treatment of 66 children with migraines. It was found to be as effective as the standard therapy but those who were given propofol had a lower rate of headache recurrence within 24 hours.

Propofol is a drug of abuse that was in part responsible for the death of Michael Jackson (it was one of several drugs found in his body). Because it is only given intravenously and is not easy to get, most of the cases of addiction reported occurred in healthcare professionals.

Propofol is administered intravenously under the supervision of an anesthesiologist. At anesthetic doses, it can have serious side effects such as a drop in blood pressure. However, it appears safe for conscious sedation. It is probably even safer at small doses used for migraines.

It can be considered when a patient does not respond to intravenous magnesium, ketorolac, metoclopramide, dexamethasone, and dihydroergotamine.

98. Hydroxyzine (3)

Please read about it in the section about preventive drugs as it is used both as an acute and preventive medication.

Opioids

The main problem with opioid or narcotic drugs is that they do not relieve migraines and can cause or worsen nausea. If taken more than once a week, opioids can also cause medication overuse (or rebound) headaches even in the absence of addiction. Regular intake of opioids can worsen other pain conditions, such as neck and back pain, by causing hyperalgesia. Hyperalgesia is an increased sensitivity to pain.

There are exceptions when occasional use of opioids is appropriate. If a patient has contraindications for the use of NSAIDs, triptans, and gepants or they are ineffective, an opioid drug can be tried. The drug should not be taken more than once a week. In the case of menstrual migraines, it can be taken daily for 3-5 days within one month.

In addition to addiction and physical dependence, opioids can cause constipation, upset stomach, dizziness, drowsiness, and other side effects.

Different opioids have a similar mechanism of action but, as with NSAIDs or triptans, they may have different effects in different patients. Some prefer codeine, others respond better to oxycodone, hydrocodone, or hydromorphone.

As a headache specialist, I tend to see many patients who have visited numerous doctors and have unsuccessfully tried various treatments. The majority of these patients do not respond to opioids either. Over the years, however, I have accumulated several dozen patients who are doing well on opioid drugs. Some even take opioids for the prevention of attacks. You can read about the preventive use of opioids in the section below.

99. Codeine (3)

Codeine is a mild opioid pain killer. It can cause addiction and can be a "gateway drug" leading to the abuse of stronger prescription and illicit drugs. Some countries allow codeine to be sold without a doctor's prescription, but it is always in combination with other drugs. In Canada, 8 mg of codeine is always mixed with two other drugs, usually with acetaminophen and caffeine. It is sold without a prescription, but from behind the counter and not from open shelves.

A combination of 30 mg of codeine with caffeine, butalbital, and either acetaminophen or aspirin (Fioricet with codeine and Fiorinal with codeine) is particularly problematic because caffeine can also cause medication overuse headache and butalbital is also addictive.

Twenty-five milligrams of codeine with 400 mg of acetaminophen is as effective as 1,000 mg of aspirin according to a 198-patient trial. Both treatments were more effective than the placebo.

100. Tramadol (3)

Tramadol (Ultram) is a mild narcotic (opioid) pain killer. Just like other opioids, it is not a good choice to treat an acute migraine attack. Besides its addiction potential, it does not work well for most migraine patients, can cause nausea, and can lead to rebound or medication overuse headaches.

Tramadol is also available in combination with acetaminophen (Ultracet). This combination was tested in a study published in *Headache*, Tramadol/Acetaminophen for the Treatment of Acute Migraine Pain: Findings of a Randomized, Placebo-Controlled Trial. 305 patients took tramadol/APAP (75 mg/650 mg) or placebo for a typical migraine with moderate or severe pain.

Subjects in the tramadol/APAP group were more likely than those in the placebo group to be pain-free at 2 hours (22% vs. 9%), 6 hours (43% vs. 25%), and 24 hours (53% vs. 38%). Side effects caused by the active drug included nausea, dizziness, vomiting, and somnolence.

The usual dose of tramadol for acute pain is 50 to 100 mg every 4 to 6 hours. The maximum daily dose is 400 mg.

101. Butorphanol* (3)

Butorphanol nasal spray (Stadol NS) is specifically approved by the FDA for the treatment of acute migraine attacks. It belongs to the so-called agonist-antagonist type of opioid drugs, while morphine, methadone, oxycodone, and most other opioids are pure agonist drugs. The agonist-antagonist drugs were originally thought to be less addictive. Unfortunately, this is not the case.

In addition to typical opioid side effects, butorphanol is more likely to cause hallucinations. I never prescribe this drug.

Anti-nausea drugs

102. Metoclopramide (5)

Metoclopramide (Reglan) is an anti-nausea drug that has been in use since 1979. Controlled studies have shown that metoclopramide stops not only nausea and vomiting that often accompany migraine attacks but also pain.

The American Headache Society (AHS) and the European Federation of Neurological Societies (EFNS) guidelines recommend intravenous metoclopramide as an effective treatment in the management of acute migraine. While intravenous (IV) administration is preferred, intramuscular (IM), subcutaneous (SC) and oral routes are also effective.

These guidelines were based on many high-quality blinded studies. One such study was done by doctors in Pennsylvania. They compared 10 mg of IV metoclopramide with 600 mg of ibuprofen. Metoclopramide was more effective.

A meta-analysis of 13 studies of intravenous metoclopramide involving 655 patients showed that "Metoclopramide is an effective treatment for migraine headache." and that "it should be considered a primary agent in the treatment of acute migraines in emergency departments".

Another emergency room study was done by doctors at the Albert Einstein College of Medicine after this meta-analysis was published. It compared IV metoclopramide with IV ketorolac and IV valproate in 330 patients. Metoclopramide was the most effective of the three.

We give IV metoclopramide in the office and prescribe it in a tablet form. However, this drug can have bothersome side effects. Drowsiness is one of the common ones. A much more unpleasant side effect is severe restlessness or akathisia. Some patients describe it as wanting to crawl out of their skin, being restless, and very uncomfortable. This side effect can be relieved by diphenhydramine given IV or as a tablet. According to a Turkish study, the incidence of this side effect is 6% if the IV infusion is given over 15 minutes and 25% if given as a "push" in under a minute. We usually give it as a "push" and find that significantly fewer than 20% of patients develop this side effect.

A much more serious side effect of metoclopramide is tardive dyskinesia or involuntary movements of the mouth, face, or another part of the body. The FDA warning states in part: "The development of this condition is directly related to the length of time a patient is taking metoclopramide and the number of doses taken. Those at greatest risk include the elderly, especially older women, and people who have been on the drug for a long time. Tardive dyskinesia is rarely reversible and there is no known treatment. However, in some patients, symptoms may lessen or resolve after metoclopramide treatment is stopped". A recent review estimates that tardive dyskinesia happens in less than 1% of patients.

This very rare but devastating side effect is not likely to occur in our patients who receive metoclopramide infrequently. However, the thought of tardive dyskinesia is always lurking in the back of our minds so we tend to use

IV ondansetron, a safer nausea drug. Since ondansetron does not help with pain, we combine it with IV ketorolac or another medication.

Metoclopramide is available in 5 and 10 mg tablets. The maximum daily dose is 60 mg.

103. Domperidone (4)

Domperidone (Motilium) is not a type of champagne. That would be Dom Perignon and it could give you a headache. It is an excellent nausea medication that is often used for the treatment of migraine-associated nausea.

Domperidone works differently from other nausea medications and can be effective when other drugs are not. Besides being good at relieving nausea, one study suggested that it can prevent migraine attacks if taken in the prodrome period, 6 to 12 hours before the attack. Prodrome is a prelude to a migraine attack and it can consist of fatigue, elation, irritability, depression, yawning, increased urination, food cravings, and others. Not every person has a prodrome, although some people are simply not aware of it since it can occur a day or two before the attack.

Doctors at the City of London Migraine Clinic conducted a rigorous study of domperidone. It showed that domperidone shortens migraine attacks when taken with paracetamol (acetaminophen). Another study by a different British group showed that a combination of domperidone with paracetamol (Domperamol) is as effective as 50 mg of sumatriptan.

A study comparing domperidone with another nausea drug, metoclopramide, showed that they are equally effective for nausea in diabetics with gastric motility problems. Domperidone, however, had fewer neurological side effects. Although domperidone has few side effects it should be used with caution in older patients. It can cause serious cardiac arrhythmias or abnormal heartbeats.

In a tablet form, the dose of domperidone is 10 mg, up to three times a day. In a suppository, the dose is 30 mg and it can be taken up to twice a day.

Domperidone is available in 58 countries but not in the US. In desperate cases, I've had some patients get it from Canada or Europe.

104. Aprepitant (3)

Aprepitant (Emend) is an anti-nausea drug that has a different mechanism of action from all other such drugs, so it can help when other medications do not help or when they cause side effects.

A study published in *Neurology* by Dr. Denise Chou and her colleagues describes the use of oral aprepitant in the treatment of DHE-induced nausea in hospitalized patients.

The authors reviewed hourly diary data and clinical notes of patients admitted to the hospital for the treatment of refractory migraine headaches (status migrainosus) with DHE infusions between 2011 and 2015.

They identified 74 such patients, 24 of whom had kept daily diaries. In 36 of 57 cases in which aprepitant was given, there was a 50% reduction in the number of other anti-nausea medications given to patients. Of 57 patients, 52 reported that the addition of aprepitant improved nausea. Among 21 of 24 patients with hourly diary data, nausea scores were reduced. In all 12 patients with vomiting, aprepitant stopped it. Aprepitant was well tolerated and caused no side effects.

The authors concluded that aprepitant can be effective in the treatment of refractory DHE-induced nausea and vomiting. They also suggested that perhaps this drug could be used for migraine-related nausea even when DHE is not given.

It is available in 40, 80, and 125 mg tablets.

Phenothiazines

Phenothiazines were originally developed for schizophrenia. Later they were found to be effective for the treatment of nausea. They can relieve not only nausea that accompanies migraine but the pain as well.

Side effects of phenothiazine drugs include drowsiness, dizziness, akathisia, or restlessness. Akathisia or restlessness is a most unpleasant side effect. It is also seen with metoclopramide and is described above. This side effect can be relieved by diphenhydramine. Prolonged use of phenothiazines can lead to persistent involuntary movements, which are also described under metoclopramide.

105. Chlorpromazine (3)

Chlorpromazine (Thorazine) was the first drug in the family of phenothiazines. It was approved for the treatment of schizophrenia in 1950. Phenothiazine drugs have also been found to be effective for the treatment of nausea and vomiting, severe anxiety, and persistent hiccups.

The Australian & New Zealand Association of Neurologists recommends chlorpromazine as one of the drugs for the treatment of moderate to severe migraine in an emergency setting.

Chlorpromazine is approved by the FDA for the treatment of schizophrenia, severe mania, nausea, vomiting, severe hiccups, and other conditions. Chlorpromazine is considered to be stronger than other phenothiazines, but it can have more side effects. Side effects include dizziness, drowsiness, blurred vision, and others. A higher incidence of side effects is why chlorpromazine is used for nausea only if milder drugs such as ondansetron, metoclopramide, and prochlorperazine do not help.

The usual dose of chlorpromazine for nausea is 10 or 25 mg taken up to four times a day.

106. Prochlorperazine (5)

Prochlorperazine (Compazine) is another phenothiazine drug. It is mostly used for the treatment of nausea and vomiting and it is available in tablets, rectal suppositories, and injections. According to an Iranian study, prochlorperazine appears to be an effective drug not only for the treatment of nausea and vomiting associated with migraine but also for head pain and other symptoms.

Prochlorperazine was found to be more effective in treating all migraine symptoms than another antiemetic (nausea drug), metoclopramide. In a study of children with migraine seen in an emergency department, intravenous prochlorperazine was more effective than an intravenous pain medication ketorolac.

I do have patients for whom chlorpromazine works exceptionally well and with no side effects. Most of them need it not more than a few times a month and most use tablets and less often, suppositories. Suppositories work faster than tablets and are preferred by patients who experience vomiting with their migraines.

The usual dose is 5 or 10 mg by mouth up to four times a day or 25 mg by a rectal suppository, up to twice a day.

107. Promethazine (5)

Promethazine (Phenergan) is also effective for the treatment of migraine-induced nausea and vomiting. It has not been studied as extensively as prochlorperazine or metoclopramide for the treatment of migraines. A double-blind study in 216 Iranian patients comparing sumatriptan with promethazine with sumatriptan alone, showed that the combination was more effective in relieving pain, achieving a pain-free state, and preventing recurrence of migraine.

Promethazine is available in 12.5 mg, 25 mg, and 50 mg tablets and suppositories. It can be also given as an injection.

Setrons

108. Ondansetron (3)

Ondansetron (Zofran) belongs to the family of setrons. There are no good studies of ondansetron for the treatment of migraines, but the impression of most headache specialists is that it is helpful only for the treatment of nausea and not the pain of migraine. However, one large observational study by doctors at Boston Children's Hospital does suggest that in children it may help more than just nausea. Observational studies are much less reliable than double-blind placebo-controlled ones. The large size of this study, however, provides some compensation for this deficiency. The researchers looked at the records of 32,124 children with migraine who presented to the emergency room. One fifth received ondansetron and it was as effective in preventing a return visit to the ER as metoclopramide, while prochlorperazine was a bit more effective.

The advantage of ondansetron is that it does not cause neurological side effects. It can cause constipation, diarrhea, drowsiness, fatigue, and fever.

Ondansetron is available in 4 mg and 8 mg tablets, orally disintegrating tablets, and as an injection, but not as a suppository.

109. Granisetron (3)

Granisetron (Kytril, Sancuso) is approved for the prevention and treatment of chemotherapy-induced and post-surgical nausea and vomiting. It is also used to treat nausea occurring with migraine attacks.

Granisetron was found to relieve both nausea and pain in <u>one anecdotal observation of 7 patients</u> and two controlled trials. <u>The first study was conducted in Canada and it involved 28 patients who presented to the emergency department with an acute migraine</u>. This was a randomized, double-blind, placebo-controlled study of two different doses of intravenous granisetron. Statistics are not reliable in such small trials but the active groups provided better pain and nausea relief than the placebo.

The second study was also conducted in an emergency room and included 148 patients. The study compared 2 mg of intravenous granisetron with 10 mg of intravenous metoclopramide. The drugs were found to be equally effective in the treatment of nausea, but granisetron was better at relieving pain.

Granisetron is available in 1 mg tablets. 1 or 2 mg once a day is the usual dose.

Preventive Drugs

Another reminder – the number after each drug is my subjective overall score for the drug on a 1-10 scale, 10 being close to a miracle and 1 saying, don't bother. You won't find either score in this book.

Asterisk indicates that the drug or treatment is approved by the FDA or the European Medicines Agency.

CGRP monoclonal antibodies

Calcitonin gene-related peptide (CGRP) monoclonal antibodies (mAbs) were first introduced in 2018 after decades of research. They represent a true breakthrough in the preventive treatment of migraines. They are approved for the prevention of both chronic and episodic migraines.

Three of these drugs are given by an injection under the skin (subcutaneously). The fourth one is given intravenously. All four mAbs have similar rates of overall efficacy. Some patients, however, may respond better to one or another drug. This is particularly the case when switching between erenumab, a drug that blocks CGRP receptor to one of the other three drugs that bind to the CGRP molecule.

These drugs do not have any interactions with other medications and have a surprisingly low incidence of side effects. Erenumab is the only drug in this class that can cause serious constipation and elevated blood pressure. This is possibly related to its different mechanism of action.

The most common side effects of the three subcutaneous drugs are injection site reactions such as redness, pain, and swelling. Allergic reactions can also occur. Most are mild and consist of a rash. Severe ones such as an anaphylactic shock are very rare. No deaths have been reported due to any of these drugs.

The cost of all four drugs is similarly high and most US insurers will pay for them only if you first try and fail two oral preventive medications such as a blood pressure medicine, an antidepressant, or an epilepsy drug.

110. Erenumab* (5)

Erenumab (Aimovig) was the first drug in the family of mAbs against CGRP to be approved by the FDA.

Erenumab is available in an autoinjector which makes the drug easy to self-administer. Its main side effect is constipation, which at times can be severe and some patients required surgery. New onset or worsening of preexistent hypertension is another possible side effect.

The dose of erenumab is either 70 mg or 140 mg given monthly. It provides dramatic, sometimes 100%, relief to about one in five patients. About 50% of patients report a 50% decline in the frequency of attacks. It should be tried for at least two months before switching to another preventive drug.

111. Fremanezumab* (6)

Fremanezumab (Ajovy) is also approved for the preventive treatment of episodic and chronic migraine headaches.

Fremanezumab differs from erenumab and galcanezumab in that it can be injected monthly (225 mg) or every three months (675 mg).

It is available in a pre-filled syringe as well as an auto-injector.

112. Galcanezumab* (6)

Galcanezumab (Emgality) is injected monthly. The first dose is two shots or 240 mg, followed by monthly injections of 120 mg.

Galcanezumab has the distinction of being the only CGRP mAb approved for the treatment of cluster headaches. The monthly dose for cluster headaches is 300 mg.

113. Eptinezumab* (6)

Eptienzumab (Vyepti) is different from the other three drugs in that it is administered intravenously every three months. It is given by a 30-minute infusion. The monthly dose is either 100 or 300 mg.

Eptinezumab has a faster onset of action because it is administered intravenously and quickly reaches its peak concentration in the blood. The other three drugs take up to a week to reach their maximum concentration.

Eptinezumab works for patients who do not respond to the other three drugs because of a better distribution of the drug and because these four mAbs are not identical.

The most common side effect in clinical trials was nasopharyngitis or a common cold. It occurred in 6% of patients on the 100 mg dose and 8% on the 300 mg dose. It occurred in 6% of patients on placebo. This suggests that the drug was not the cause of the cold. An allergic reaction occurred in 1% to 2% of patients. It consisted of itching and flushing.

Antidepressants

Antidepressants seem to work on a range of brain chemicals or neurotransmitters. Some of these neurotransmitters are also involved in the development of migraines and pain. People who have chronic pain or migraines are more likely to develop anxiety and depression. This is not only because having chronic pain makes you depressed. The connection is bi-directional, in that if you suffer from anxiety or depression you are more likely to develop migraine headaches and other pain problems.

Many patients become offended when prescribed an antidepressant. They reasonably assume that the doctor does not believe that they have real pain. Many studies have shown that certain antidepressants relieve pain even when a person is not depressed.

In short-term studies of major depression, antidepressants increased the risk of suicidal thinking and behavior in children, adolescents, and young adults. This is less likely to occur when treating pain, but many pain patients also suffer from depression.

Tricyclic antidepressants

Tricyclic antidepressants (TCAs) are proven to relieve many different types of pain. The dose to treat migraines and pain is usually lower than the dose used to treat depression.

The side effects of TCAs include dry mouth, dizziness, weight gain, sexual dysfunction, urinary retention, and other side effects. Constipation can usually be managed with over-the-counter remedies, such as an extract of senna or polyethylene glycol.

TCAs can cause cardiac arrhythmias, especially at high doses. In people with heart disease or multiple risk factors for heart disease, an electrocardiogram should be done before starting a TCA. These drugs should be avoided in the elderly because of an increased risk of falls due to sedation and because they can cause serious constipation. Tricyclics can lower the seizure threshold and should be avoided in people with epilepsy. An overdose of any of the TCAs can be lethal.

Fluoxetine (Prozac) and similar drugs in the SSRI family have fewer side effects. They mostly replaced the TCAs for the treatment of depression. However, SSRIs do not help pain or headaches, so the TCAs remain popular for the treatment of pain and headaches.

114. Amitriptyline (5)

Amitriptyline (Elavil) was approved in the US in 1961 for depression.

Several controlled trials have proven the efficacy of amitriptyline in the prevention of migraines.

Amitriptyline can also relieve insomnia. On the other hand, in some people, the sedating effect lasts too long and they feel sleepy or tired the next day. If that happens, it is worth trying a different TCA that could be less sedating. Because of possible excessive sedation, this and most other preventive drugs are started at a small dose. For amitriptyline, it is 10 or 25 mg nightly. For some, 25 mg is all they need. Others may require 100 mg or more. This is often due to the variable absorption of the drug. Fortunately, the absorption of amitriptyline can be assessed by a blood test. The test is not necessary if the medicine is working. If a patient has no relief and no side effects at a 100 mg dose, I check their blood level. If the level is low, it is safe to continue increasing the dose. The official maximum daily dose is 300 mg.

115. Nortriptyline (5)

Nortriptyline (Pamelor) is also approved by the FDA only for the treatment of depression.

Nortriptyline is similar to amitriptyline. It tends to cause fewer and milder side effects. This could be because amitriptyline is broken down in the body into nortriptyline. Nortriptyline is the active form of amitriptyline.

There are no good blinded studies of nortriptyline for the prevention of migraines and they are not likely to be done. We assume it is as good as amitriptyline, although studies of amitriptyline also lack in size and scientific rigor.

Trials of nortriptyline for various pain conditions were done years ago and they do not meet our modern standards.

Pain and headaches sometimes respond to as little as 10 or 25 mg. As with amitriptyline, blood levels of nortriptyline can be useful at higher doses. The maximum daily dose is 150 mg.

116. Desipramine (4)

Desipramine (Norpramin) is used much less frequently for migraines than amitriptyline or nortriptyline. There are no controlled trials of this drug for the prevention of migraines. However, it has been proven to be as effective in relieving the pain of diabetic neuropathy as amitriptyline. It was also shown to be effective for the treatment of postherpetic neuralgia (shingles pain) and chronic low back pain.

Desipramine has the advantage of being less sedating and causing fewer other side effects, such as dry mouth and constipation. In one study, desipramine caused less weight gain than amitriptyline (but as much as nortriptyline). The dose is 10 or 25 mg nightly with a gradual increase as needed and as tolerated. The maximum daily dose is 300 mg.

117. Protriptyline (4)

Protriptyline (Vivactil) also causes less sleepiness than amitriptyline. It has never been subjected to clinical trials for migraines. If someone, however, has good relief on another TCA but drowsiness or another side effect is a problem, protriptyline may help with fewer side effects.

The starting dose of protriptyline is 10 mg nightly and after a couple of weeks, it is increased to 20 mg and then, to a maximum of 30 mg.

SSRIs

The SSRI category of antidepressants became popular not because these drugs were more effective than the older antidepressants, but because they had fewer side effects. SSRIs can cause side effects. These include nausea, dizziness, insomnia, loss of libido, inability to reach an orgasm, and other symptoms.

SSRIs were also studied for various painful conditions but were not found to be effective. They do help some patients. This could be due to the placebo effect or because the relief of anxiety and depression may indirectly help migraine headaches and pain.

An <u>authoritative Cochrane review of published studies</u> of SSRIs for the prevention of migraines found that "Over 2 months of treatment, SSRIs are no more efficacious than placebo in patients with migraine."

118. Fluoxetine (3)

Fluoxetine (Prozac, Sarafem), the first drug in the family of selective serotonin reuptake inhibitors (SSRIs), was introduced in 1986.

<u>One study of 32 patients showed that fluoxetine was effective for the prevention of migraines</u> without relieving depression. Another <u>52-patient trial also found a positive effect that was not accompanied by</u> an improvement in depression. However, a more rigorous and larger 122-patient study <u>showed no effect of fluoxetine on migraines</u>.

One advantage of fluoxetine compared to other antidepressants is its long half-life. This means that stopping it suddenly rarely causes unpleasant withdrawal symptoms.

The usual dose of fluoxetine is 20 mg and the maximum dose is 80 mg.

SNRIs

Unlike SSRIs, selective norepinephrine-serotonin inhibitors (SNRIs) treat not only depression and anxiety but also relieve pain and prevent migraine headaches. . A review of studies that involved a total of 418 patients showed that SNRIs are effective for the prevention of migraines.

Potential side effects include insomnia, drowsiness, fatigue, nausea, dizziness, suicidal thoughts in depressed children and young adults, and others.

Sudden discontinuation of SNRIs can cause withdrawal symptoms. These may include one or more of the following: dizziness, headache, nausea, diarrhea, paresthesia (pins-and-needles), irritability, vomiting, insomnia, anxiety, sweating, and fatigue. SNRIs are stopped after a slow and gradual reduction in the dose.

119. Venlafaxine (4)

Venlafaxine (Effexor), the first SNRI, was approved by the FDA for depression in 1993. Venlafaxine works as an SSRI at low doses and as an SNRI at doses higher than 75 mg a day.

The 150 mg dose was more effective than 75 mg in a 60-patient trial. A double-blind crossover study comparing venlafaxine with amitriptyline showed them to be equally effective. Venlafaxine had fewer side effects than amitriptyline.

Venlafaxine is considered to be effective at a dose of 150 mg, but it is started at 75 mg. After a week or two, the dose is increased to 150 mg. The maximum daily dose of venlafaxin is 450 mg.

120. Duloxetine (5)

Duloxetine (Cymbalta) is approved by the FDA for the treatment of major depression, generalized anxiety, musculoskeletal pain, such as low back pain, and pain due to osteoarthritis, fibromyalgia, and diabetic peripheral neuropathy. Unlike venlafaxine, its dual mechanism of action is present at the lowest dose.

Duloxetine is not approved for the treatment of migraine headaches, but it is widely used for this indication. Because duloxetine relieves different types of pain, it is likely to help migraines as well. It is a particularly good choice in patients who also have anxiety and depression. These two conditions are 2-3 times more likely to occur in migraine sufferers.

Several small studies show that duloxetine may be effective for chronic migraines with medication overuse. Most migraine studies used 60 mg a day.

One small study suggests that 120 mg is more effective for the prevention of episodic migraine headaches.

The starting dose of duloxetine is 20 or 30 mg. After a couple of weeks, the dose can be increased to 60 mg. Only a few of my patients have gone up to 120 mg.

121. Desvenlafaxine (4)

Desvenlafaxine (Pristiq) is a derivative of venlafaxine. Venlafaxine is broken down in the body into its active form, desvenlafaxine. Desvenlafaxine can be considered a purified form of venlafaxine. The FDA-recommended starting and maintenance dose of desvenlafaxine is 50 mg daily. Some patients may need to take 100 mg.

There are no published studies of desvenlafaxine for migraine headaches. However, considering that two other SNRI drugs, duloxetine and milnacipran relieve pain, it is likely that desvenlafaxine can also work for pain and migraines.

122. Milnacipran (4)

Milnacipran (Savella) is similar to other SNRIs. It is approved by the FDA only for the treatment of fibromyalgia. Fibromyalgia is a chronic disorder characterized by widespread musculoskeletal pain, fatigue, and tenderness in localized areas. Fibromyalgia, back pain, and other pains are more common in people with migraines. This means that if you have one type of pain, you are more likely to have another.

The manufacturer of milnacipran decided not to seek approval for the treatment of depression to avoid the stigma of antidepressants. Many patients feel that if they are prescribed an antidepressant, their pain is not perceived as real physical pain, but purely psychological.

Milnacipran was tested for the preventive treatment of migraines in one unblinded observational study. Not surprisingly, it was effective.

The usual dose of milnacipran is 50 mg twice a day. The maximum dose is 100 mg twice a day.

MAOI

123. Phenelzine (3)

Phenelzine (Nardil) was approved by the FDA for the treatment of depression in 1961. It belongs to the family of monoamine oxidase inhibitors (MAOIs) and it is an effective antidepressant. However, it is rarely used because it causes more side effects than other antidepressants and can have serious drug and food interactions.

There have been no good trials of phenelzine for the treatment of migraines. One small study compared phenelzine with and without a beta-blocker, atenolol. Atenolol is known to help migraines and lowers blood pressure, so it could prevent an increase in blood pressure from phenelzine. Phenelzine worked well with and without atenolol. Another report described the use of phenelzine in 11 patients with migraines who did not respond to several drugs. Ten of the 11 patients had a greater than 50% reduction in the number of headache attacks. Two patients developed low blood pressure. One patient developed high blood pressure, which was easily controlled. There is also a case report of dramatic improvement in a patient with chronic and treatment-resistant migraine.

Phenelzine can interact with other antidepressants, appetite suppressants, drugs for attention deficit disorder, some epilepsy drugs, muscle relaxants, certain blood pressure medications, opioid medications, and others. Foods that can interact with phenelzine include aged, dried, fermented, salted, smoked, pickled, and processed meats and fish, aged cheeses, fava beans, Italian green beans, broad beans, overripe or spoiled fruits, packaged soups, sauerkraut, red wine, and some other types of alcohol.

An interaction with these drugs and foods can cause a sudden increase in blood pressure and serotonin syndrome. Both conditions can be dangerous. However, it does not mean that every drug and food listed above will always cause a serious reaction. Most people will have a mild or no reaction at all. If another drug needs to be added to phenelzine, it can be started at a low dose, and then the dose can be slowly increased.

Besides drug and food interactions, phenelzine can have unpleasant side effects of its own. These include drowsiness, dizziness, constipation, dry mouth, weight gain, sexual dysfunction, and others.

I prescribe phenelzine only after trying many other preventive drugs. In some patients, it works exceptionally well. The starting and maintenance dose is 15 mg three times a day.

Other psychotropics

124. Mirtazapine (3)

Mirtazapine (Remeron) is a tetracyclic antidepressant similar to TCAs. Just like TCAs, it has pain-relieving properties.

The analgesic properties of mirtazapine are much less proven than those of TCAs. Only anecdotal reports have suggested that it is effective in the preventive treatment of migraine headaches. In a small but well-conducted double-blind trial, it provided good relief of tension-type headaches. A single case report described a patient whose cluster headaches consistently responded to mirtazapine.

Mirtazapine has similar side effects to TCAs but they are usually milder. It can cause drowsiness and is best taken at night. Other potential side effects are dizziness, weight gain, constipation, and dry mouth.

The starting dose of mirtazapine is 15 mg. It can be increased up to 45 mg a day. The same dose can be effective for depression and pain.

125. Clonazepam (2)

Clonazepam (Klonopin) is approved for the treatment of panic attacks and certain types of seizures. It is also used "off-label" to treat anxiety, insomnia, and muscle spasm. Clonazepam belongs to the family of benzodiazepines. This class includes diazepam (Valium), alprazolam (Xanax), and lorazepam (Ativan). Clonazepam tends to have a longer-lasting effect. It is thought to be less likely to cause physical and psychological dependence and tolerance, although this is not proven. Tolerance means that the drug loses its efficacy over time and to maintain the effect the dose has to be continuously increased.

Clonazepam is rarely used alone to treat migraine headaches. Combining clonazepam with other medications, however, can provide additional relief. This could be in part because patients with migraines are more likely to have anxiety and panic attacks. They also often live in fear of their next migraine. This anxiety and tension can lead to a self-fulfilling prophecy. One anecdotal report details stories of three patients who greatly benefited from clonazepam after they did not respond to a variety of other treatments.

I prescribe it very infrequently and usually to patients in whom anxiety, neck pain, or insomnia are major contributors to their migraine headaches and who do not improve with other treatments.

126. Buspirone (2)

Antidepressants are proven to relieve anxiety even in the absence of depression. They are a better long-term solution than anxiety drugs such as diazepam or alprazolam because antidepressants are not addictive and do not lose their efficacy over time. A unique drug that is used only for anxiety and not depression and that does not cause addiction, is buspirone (Buspar).

Several studies suggest that buspirone is effective for the treatment of migraines. A 74-patient double-blind, placebo-controlled study showed a 43% reduction in headache frequency in the buspirone-treated group, but only a 10% reduction in the placebo group. This effect was independent of the presence or absence of anxiety.

Buspirone has a fairly benign side effect profile and does not cause withdrawal symptoms when stopped suddenly. This is a common problem with other anxiety drugs and many antidepressants.

The starting dose is 7.5 mg twice a day. The maximum dose is 30 mg twice a day.

Epilepsy drugs

People with epilepsy are more likely to have migraines and vice versa. Sometimes it is difficult to differentiate migraine aura from a small epileptic event, a so-called partial complex seizure.

Epilepsy drugs stop seizures by reducing the excessive excitability of neurons, or brain cells. Since certain neurons in migraine patients are also hyperexcitable, it is not surprising that anti-epilepsy drugs can prevent migraines.

127. Valproate* (4)

Valproate (Depakote) was approved by the FDA in 1983 to treat epilepsy, in 1985 for bipolar disorder, and 1986, for migraines.

Potential side effects include nausea, drowsiness, dizziness, hand tremor, weight gain, and hair loss.

The drug carries a so-called black box warning about potentially serious liver damage which usually occurs during the first 6 months of treatment. The FDA recommends close monitoring of patients with regular blood tests. Fatal cases of pancreatitis have also been reported. Another major problem with this drug is birth defects. It is contraindicated in pregnancy. The majority of migraine sufferers are women of child-bearing age and up to half of the pregnancies in the US are unplanned. This and all of the other potential side effects is why I rarely prescribe valproate. The other side effects include weight gain, hair loss, dizziness, drowsiness, nausea, and others.

It is reasonable to try valproate in a patient who also suffers from epilepsy or a mood disorder or who does not respond to a variety of other treatments. I advise sexually active women of child-bearing age to use two complementary methods of contraception while on valproate.

Valproate is effective for about 50% of migraine sufferers. The starting dose is 500 mg of the extended-release formulation once a day. Some patients require 1,000 mg. For epilepsy, the dose goes up to 2,000 and higher, depending on the blood level of the drug.

128. Topiramate* (5)

Topiramate (Topamax) is one of the most popular preventive drugs for migraine. This is not because it is more effective than other approved drugs. It is because it can cause weight loss. The drug manufacturer tried to get it approved for weight loss. The FDA, however, felt that while the cognitive side effects may be acceptable when treating epilepsy or migraines, they are not acceptable when treating obesity.

Cognitive side effects can be obvious to most patients but for some, they are not. People begin to attribute their memory and word-finding difficulties to stress, lack of sleep, early-onset dementia, and other reasons. They have told me that they feel stupid on this drug. Topiramate can also cause irritability, depression, fatigue, osteoporosis, glaucoma, and in 20%, kidney stones (10% with symptoms and 10% without). Like valproate, it is contraindicated in pregnancy because it can cause birth defects. I urge patients taking this drug to be vigilant about contraception.

In clinical trials, 55% of patients had relief and were able to tolerate the drug. The starting dose of topiramate is 25 mg nightly with a weekly increase of 25 mg up to 100 mg. Occasionally, patients benefit from a higher dose, up to 200 mg. If cognitive side effects are mild but bothersome, it may be worth trying a long-acting form of topiramate which can have fewer side effects. There are two such products on the market in the US. They are much more expensive than generic topiramate.

Topiramate is also approved for migraines in adolescents, ages 12 to 17. In this age group, it can cause or worsen an eating disorder.

129. Zonisamide (3)

Zonisamide (Zonegran) is an epilepsy drug similar to topiramate in its mechanism of action. Unfortunately, it shares its side effects as well. These include fatigue, difficulty with concentration and memory, nausea, and others. However, because they are not identical drugs, some patients tolerate zonisamide better than topiramate.

One study showed that 44% of 172 patients who did not respond to topiramate did respond to zonisamide with 13% having an excellent response. A similar study of 63 patients who did not respond to topiramate also showed improvement from zonisamide as did 34 patients in another study. Zonisamide also helped 8 out of 12 children who did not respond to other medications.

The dose of zonisamide ranges from 50 to 400 mg a day, but most patients need 100-200 mg.

130. Gabapentin (3)

Gabapentin (Neurontin) is a drug that was originally developed for the treatment of epilepsy. Now it is used for many neurological conditions but rarely for epilepsy. It is usually not strong enough to stop epileptic seizures. Gabapentin can relieve various pain conditions, including sciatic pain, and it has an official FDA approval for the treatment of postherpetic neuralgia, or shingles pain.

Gabapentin can help some patients with episodic and chronic migraines. However, a review of five clinical trials of gabapentin for the treatment of episodic migraine found no evidence that it works. The authors of the review concluded that "Since adverse events were common among the gabapentin-treated patients, it is advocated that gabapentin should not be used in routine clinical practice". The adverse effects were mostly dizziness and somnolence.

Because gabapentin is proven to relieve painful conditions and because it has a relatively benign side effect profile, I prescribe it for some patients with episodic and chronic migraine. It can also help patients with insomnia, although this indication is also not proven in large trials.

The dose of gabapentin can go up to 3,600 mg a day and higher. There have been some reports of gabapentin abuse and dependence at doses above 3,000 mg a day. The usual starting dose is 300 mg once or twice a day with a slow escalation as needed and as tolerated up to about 1,800 mg a day. Some patients report good relief of insomnia with 300 mg taken at night. Transition to menopause can be accompanied by temporary worsening of migraine headaches. Gabapentin can help relieve menopausal hot flashes and improve sleep at a dose of 900 mg a day.

131. Pregabalin (2)

Pregabalin (Lyrica) is an epilepsy drug that is also approved by the FDA for the treatment of neuropathic or nerve pain associated with diabetes, spinal cord injury, shingles (herpes zoster), and fibromyalgia. It has a low risk of addiction and abuse. For illicit use, it is often combined with other drugs.

Common side effects of pregabalin include dizziness, drowsiness, difficulty thinking, weight gain, sexual dysfunction, and dry mouth.

There are no large controlled trials of pregabalin for migraines. In one open-label trial, it was given to 47 migraine patients with good results. This was not a rigorous study which means that its results are not reliable. However, because it is proven to relieve other types of pain, it is also prescribed for migraines. I've seen very few patients who benefited from pregabalin without having significant side effects.

The usual starting dose is 50 mg twice a day and the maximum dose is 300 mg twice a day.

132. Lamotrigine (2)

Lamotrigine (Lamictal) is an epilepsy drug that is also approved as a mood stabilizer in bipolar disorders.

There are no good controlled trials of lamotrigine in migraines, but some reports suggest that 100 mg of lamotrigine is <u>effective not only in reducing the frequency of migraines but also in reducing the frequency and the duration of visual auras</u>. There are also case reports of <u>lamotrigine relieving complicated auras with visual and sensory symptoms</u>.

The main side effects of lamotrigine are dizziness, drowsiness, upset stomach, and rash. The rash can be serious and in rare cases fatal (Stevens-Johnson syndrome), but it could be avoided by starting with a low dose (25 mg) and increasing it by 25 mg every two weeks. For epilepsy, the dose goes up to as high as 600 mg a day.

Blood pressure drugs

Blood vessels are intricately involved in the migraine process. However, we no longer call migraines vascular headaches because brain cells begin the process and changes in the size of blood vessels come later. Like with epilepsy drugs and antidepressants, it is not clear why blood pressure medications help prevent migraines. It is even more surprising that blood pressure drugs with different mechanisms of action can prevent migraines.

Beta-blockers

These are effective drugs that were first approved for the treatment of high blood pressure. In people with normal blood pressure, they produce a minimal drop in pressure. In some, however, even a small pressure drop can cause side effects such as fatigue, weakness, lightheadedness, and fainting. These drugs also slow down the heart rate. This can make it difficult to exercise. Propranolol and timolol can worsen pre-existing asthma but newer, so-called cardioselective beta-blockers such as bisoprolol, metoprolol, and nebivolol do not. Other side effects of beta-blockers include diarrhea, constipation, cold hands and feet, depression, and sexual dysfunction.

A beta-blocker is particularly a good option for people with rapid heartbeat or anxiety. They help physical but not mental manifestations of anxiety – sweating, shaky knees and voice, and fast heart rate. Beta-blockers are proven to help performance anxiety and some people take them in small doses before giving a speech, presentation, or musical performance.

133. Propranolol* (6)

Propranolol (Inderal) was approved by the FDA in 1967 for the treatment of high blood pressure. About a decade later, it became the first drug to be approved for the preventive treatment of migraine headaches. Propranolol is also used for essential tremor, performance anxiety, fast heartbeat (tachycardia), angina, and other conditions. In 1988, British scientist Sir James Black was awarded the Nobel Prize for the discovery of propranolol.

A typical starting dose of propranolol is 60 mg of the long-acting formulation. The dose is then increased to 80, 120, and 160 mg, if needed and if tolerated.

134. Timolol* (6)

Timolol (Blocadren), is the second of the two beta-blockers approved by the FDA for the prevention of migraines. Despite having this approval, relatively few studies examined its efficacy. One study showed that it is as effective as propranolol.

The usual dose is 10 mg twice a day.

135. Metoprolol (6)

Metoprolol (Toprol) is one of the three beta-blockers (the other two are propranolol and timolol) that are included in the American Academy of Neurology guidelines for the preventive treatment of migraines.

A large double-blind study showed that metoprolol (200 mg/day) was more effective than aspirin (300 mg/day) in achieving 50% migraine frequency reduction (45% vs 30%). No significant side effects were reported in either group.

The usual starting dose is 100 mg and the maximum dose is 400 mg a day.

136. Bisoprolol (6)

Bisoprolol (Zebeta) is another beta-blocker that has scientific evidence supporting its use in migraines. A blinded study comparing 5 mg of bisoprolol with 100 mg of metoprolol, showed them to be equally effective in the treatment of migraines.

The European Federation of Neurological Societies recommends bisoprolol as a second-line beta-blocker for the prophylactic treatment of migraine headaches, after propranolol and metoprolol. The US guidelines place bisoprolol further down the list.

The starting dose is 5 mg and the dose can be gradually increased to 20 mg.

137. Nebivolol (7)

Nebivolol (Bystolic) has the advantage of having fewer side effects than other beta-blockers. It causes lower rates of fatigue, shortness of breath, and erectile dysfunction.

Nebivolol may have additional beneficial effects on the endothelium (blood vessel lining). It may also improve glucose metabolism by improving insulin sensitivity and other functions.

The usual starting dose is 5 mg and the dose can be gradually increased to 20 mg.

Angiotensin-Converting Enzyme inhibitors (ACEIs) and ACE receptor blockers (ARBs)

A review of a large database of prescriptions showed that patients taking ACEIs or ARBs were getting 50% fewer prescriptions for abortive migraine drugs than those taking a diuretic, another common drug to treat hypertension.

The advantage of ACE inhibitors and ARBs over beta-blockers is that they do not lower the heart rate, which can make exercise difficult. Both can cause fatigue and dizziness due to the lowering of blood pressure. But the weight gain and depression, occasionally seen with propranolol does not happen with ACEIs and ARBs. On the other hand, beta-blockers can sometimes help reduce anxiety. ACEIs, but not ARBs, can cause a persistent dry cough that is not dose-dependent.

138. Lisinopril (3)

Lisinopril (Prinivil, Zestril), an ACEI at 20 mg a day was shown to be effective in the prevention of migraine headaches in a double-blind cross-over study of 60 patients. Three patients stopped the drug due to cough.

An open-label study of 5 mg of lisinopril in 21 patients also showed positive results. Three patients stopped it because of a cough.

139. Candesartan (4)

Candesartan (Atacand), an ARB, prevented migraine headaches in a 60-patient Norwegian trial published in *JAMA* in 2003. This was a double-blind crossover study. This means that half of the patients were first placed on placebo and then switched to candesartan while the second group started on candesartan and then were switched to placebo. This trial showed that when compared to placebo, 16 mg of candesartan resulted in a significant reduction in the mean number of days with headache, hours with headache, days with migraine, hours with migraine, headache severity index, level of disability, and sick leave days. Candesartan was well-tolerated – there was no difference in side effects in patients taking the drug and those taking the placebo.

In another study, Norwegian researchers compared candesartan to placebo and propranolol. This 72-patient trial compared 16 mg of candesartan with placebo and with 160 mg of propranolol. Candesartan and propranolol were equally effective in reducing migraine days per month and both were significantly more effective than the placebo.

The starting dose of candesartan is usually 8 mg with escalation to 32 mg, if needed and if tolerated.

140. Telmisartan (3)

German researchers conducted a rigorous 95-patient double-blind study of telmisartan (Micardis) for the prevention of migraines. They showed that taking 80 mg of telmisartan daily was very effective. The side effects of the drug were comparable to placebo.

Telmisartan was also effective in 33 Japanese patients who did not respond to a calcium channel blocker used for the prevention of migraines.

The starting dose of telmisartan is 40 mg, once a day. It can be increased to 80 mg.

Calcium channel blockers

These drugs regulate blood vessel activity. They can also affect calcium channels in the central nervous system if the drug crosses the blood-brain barrier. Verapamil does not cross this barrier but flunarizine and cinnarizine do. These two drugs also have anti-dopamine, anti-serotonin, and antihistamine effects which could contribute to their beneficial effect. However, <u>cinnarizine and flunarizine increase the risk of parkinsonism in older people especially those who suffered a stroke or have diabetes, according to a study from Taiwan.</u>

141. Verapamil (3)

Verapamil (Calan, Isoptin) is an effective drug for the prevention of cluster headaches. It is sometimes used for migraines as well. However, the evidence for its efficacy is weak. A <u>double-blind crossover trial of 320 mg of verapamil conducted by Dr. Glen Solomon and his colleagues in Ohio in 12 migraine patients was positive</u>. Other small studies also suggested that it might help some patients.

Verapamil has a reputation among headache specialists as being effective for the prevention of frequent migraine auras and other neurological symptoms that occur with migraine attacks. This is based only on anecdotal reports – no controlled trials have been done.

The starting dose of verapamil is 120 mg a day with a possible escalation up to 480 mg. In cluster headaches, the starting dose is 240 mg and the maximum dose is as high as 960 mg. Verapamil can cause arrhythmia (irregular heartbeat), especially at higher doses. I recommend an electrocardiogram before increasing the dose above 240 mg, especially in older people.

The two most common side effects of verapamil are constipation and swelling of the feet. In some of my patients, constipation was severe and resistant to treatment. They had to stop taking the drug.

142. Cinnarizine (4)

Cinnarizine (Stugeron, Stunarone, Arlevert, Diznil) is both a calcium channel blocker and an antihistamine drug. It is not available in the US or Canada but is included in <u>some European migraine treatment guidelines</u>. It is thought to promote cerebral blood flow and has been used to treat strokes, posttraumatic symptoms, and cerebral arteriosclerosis. In the UK it is approved for "Disorders of balance - maintenance therapy for symptoms of labyrinthine disorders, including vertigo, tinnitus, nystagmus, nausea, and vomiting such as is seen in Meniere's Disease. Prophylaxis of motion sickness." It is <u>often prescribed for vertigo of central (brain) or peripheral (inner ear) origin</u> in other countries as well. Its side effects include drowsiness, sweating, dry mouth, and gastrointestinal problems.

The side effects of cinnarizine include drowsiness, sweating, dry mouth, gastrointestinal problems, and others.

The usual dose is 75 mg a day.

143. Flunarizine* (4)

Flunarizine (Sibelium) is a calcium channel blocker approved for the preventive treatment of migraines in most countries, except for the US and Japan. In many countries, flunarizine is considered to be a first-line drug for the prevention of migraines.

It is <u>as effective as propranolol.</u> In a study by Taiwanese doctors, 10 mg of <u>flunarizine was found to be more effective than 50 mg of topiramate, although</u> <u>the average dose of topiramate for migraines is 100 mg.</u> It can take 6 to 8 weeks before flunarizine becomes effective.

<u>One observational study by Indian neurologists suggested that flunarizine</u> <u>may also improve attacks of vertigo in vestibular migraine.</u> Vestibular migraine is described at the end of the book.

The two most common side effects of flunarizine are drowsiness and weight gain. It can also cause nausea, anxiety, depression, insomnia, dry mouth, and parkinsonism. I've recommended purchasing flunarizine abroad to a few of my patients who exhausted other options. None have remained on it, either because of side effects or lack of efficacy. Because these were patients who failed to respond to many other drugs, it is not surprising that they did not respond to this one either. The logistical difficulties in getting flunarizine from outside the US is another reason I stopped recommending flunarizine.

Non-steroidal anti-inflammatory drugs

Non-steroidal anti-inflammatory drugs (NSAIDs) sold without a prescription are the most popular class of drugs used to treat migraines. Inflammation is a documented part of the migraine process which explains their high efficacy. For some, aspirin is the magic bullet, for others, even a prescription-strength NSAID is ineffective. This is because the underlying genetics and brain mechanisms of migraine differ from patient to patient.

Precautions about NSAIDs are described earlier in this book, in the section on abortive drugs.

144. Aspirin (4)

A review of eight studies that included 28,326 participants concluded that regular intake of aspirin prevents migraines. What is not clear is how much to take. The effective dose is probably between 1,300 mg to 4,550 mg a week.

Aspirin prevents migraines with aura, according to Italian researchers from Turin. They reported on 194 consecutive patients who had migraine with aura and who were placed on a prophylactic medication. Ninety of these patients were on 300 mg of aspirin daily and the rest were given propranolol, topiramate, and other preventive medications. At the end of 32 weeks of observation 86% of those on aspirin had at least a 50% reduction in the frequency of attacks of migraine with aura compared with their baseline frequency. And 41% had even better results – at least a 75% reduction. In contrast, only 46% of patients on other drugs had a 50% improvement in frequency. The probability of success with aspirin was six times greater than with any other prophylactic medication, according to the lead author, Dr. Lidia Savi.

Aspirin reduces the risk of episodic migraines becoming chronic. It does not cause medication overuse headaches.

So, how does one decide whether to take aspirin for the prevention of migraines? The decision is easier if you have another reason to take it, such as coronary or cerebrovascular disease or a family history of cancer. Yes, aspirin is highly effective in preventing cancer. If you have a history of gastritis or peptic ulcers, bleeding disorder, or allergy to aspirin, the decision is also easy – don't take it. If none of the above applies to you and you are in good general health, it may be worth trying aspirin, especially if you had no relief from other preventive treatments.

145. Naproxen (4)

Naproxen was proven effective for the prevention of migraine attacks in a double-blind study by Dr. K.M.A. Welch and his colleagues. In another double-blind study by Italian researchers, 550 mg of naproxen taken twice a day prevented menstrual migraines. It also helped relieve premenstrual pain. Naproxen is rarely used for the long-term prevention of migraines because of the risk of stomach ulcers and stomach bleeding.

Other drugs

146. Acetazolamide (3)

Acetazolamide (Diamox) is a diuretic, or water pill, which is used to treat mountain sickness. Unlike other diuretics, it is selective in removing extra fluid from the brain and the lungs, rather than equally from all parts of the body.

Migraines can be triggered by traveling to high altitudes. Acetazolamide can sometimes prevent these attacks. Take it the day before the ascent and then throughout the stay at high altitude. A handful of my patients continued to take acetazolamide even after they returned to sea level because they found it to be effective in preventing all of their migraines. Most of these patients were also sensitive to barometric pressure changes. For most people, it is not necessary to take acetazolamide daily. They can prevent an attack by taking the drug the day barometric pressure drops.

To avoid having to constantly watch the weather forecast, you can set up a google alert or use WeatherX app that sends you a warning whenever barometric pressure drops. The default setting is a drop of 20 millibars of pressure. Some people are more or less sensitive to the pressure drop and the alert can be adjusted accordingly. The WeatherX company also sells earplugs to go with their app. It is not clear if putting in earplugs when the barometric pressure drops prevents migraines.

Interestingly, people who live at high altitudes, specifically in Nepal, tend to have more migraines than those living at sea level.

Acetazolamide is also used to treat headaches due to increased intracranial pressure (pressure inside the skull).

Acetazolamide is available in 125 mg, 250 mg, and an extended-release, 500 mg tablets. The usual starting dose is 250 mg once a day. Potential side effects include tingling of your face and extremities, dizziness, and an unpleasant taste of carbonated beverages. With long-term daily use, kidney stones can develop.

147. Tizanidine (3)

Tizanidine (Zanaflex) is a muscle relaxant that has been shown to relieve chronic migraines in a 200-patient double-blind study by Dr. Joel Saper and his colleagues. It may be particularly effective in people with neck and shoulder pain. The majority of migraine sufferers have such muscle pains. It is also a good choice when you have insomnia along with migraines.

The main side effects of tizanidine are drowsiness and dizziness. This is why it is usually taken at night. The starting dose is 4 mg. It can be gradually increased to 8, and then 12 mg. In the double-blind study, the median dose was 18 mg. Some patients went up to 24 mg with 8 mg taken three times a day. Very few of my patients can take that much tizanidine during the day. At most, they will take 2-4 mg twice during the day and a higher dose at night.

148. Clopidogrel (2)

Clopidogrel (Plavix) is an anticoagulant or a blood thinner. Its role in treating migraine headaches is still being worked out.

Patients who suffer from migraines, especially those who have auras, have a higher incidence of a persistent opening between the left and the right side of their heart. The opening is called patent foramen ovale or PFO. PFO is found in 25% of the general population. In most, it is small and causes no symptoms. When it is large, it can cause symptoms and needs to be closed.

Unfortunately, studies that are aimed to relieve migraines by closing the PFO did not show much benefit. However, blood thinners used after the procedure may have helped some patients. A British physician first reported relief of migraines with clopidogrel in a small group of patients. A Canadian study showed that clopidogrel with aspirin was more effective in improving migraines than aspirin alone after surgical closure of an atrial septal defect (ASD). ASD is similar to PFO. Another study by Dr. Toomas Toomsoo of Estonia, compared aspirin and clopidogrel in patients with PFO who had not undergone surgery and it found them to be equally effective in improving migraines.

In a study by two Chinese doctors, PFO was found in 151 out of 266 (57%) of migraine patients. Of these 151, 65 had a large PFO. PFO was found in 59 out of 84 (70%) of migraine patients with aura. 27 migraine patients who did not respond to standard medical therapy were given clopidogrel, 75 mg a day for 3 months. 22 patients completed this study. Headache frequency, severity, and duration were significantly decreased by the addition of this drug. Migraine-related disability was also reduced.

Aspirin, clopidogrel, prasugrel (Effient), and ticagrelor (Brilinta) are drugs that inhibit the function of platelets, small blood particles that are involved in blood clotting. Platelet dysfunction and other blood clotting problems have been suspected to play a role in triggering migraines, but the scientific evidence has been lacking.

Cardiologist Dr. Robert Sommer and his colleagues at the Columbia University Medical Center reviewed records of their 136 patients with PFO. Migraines improved on clopidogrel in 80 (59%). The clopidogrel was equally beneficial in patients with episodic and chronic migraines, with and without aura. When the researchers tested platelets in non-responders, 19 of 45 (40%) did not have their platelets inhibited by clopidogrel. Sixteen of those patients were switched to prasugrel, which adequately inhibited platelets and 10 of 16 (62%) had improvement in their migraines. Fifty-six of 90 responders had their PFO closed and the drug stopped after three months, which is typically done after a PFO closure. Ninety-four percent had ongoing migraine relief. All eight of eight responders who stopped their medication without PFO closure had a worsening of their migraines.

This was not a blinded study, so it is premature to recommend PFO closure to migraine patients. However, patients whose migraines do not respond to the usual treatments may need to have an echocardiogram to look for a PFO. If one is found, a trial of clopidogrel is a reasonable approach.

149. Memantine (2)

Memantine (Namenda) is an Alzheimer's drug that has been used for the treatment of pain and migraine headaches. This drug blocks the NMDA receptor in the brain, which is involved in the processing of pain messages and other neurological conditions such as epilepsy, stroke, and traumatic brain injuries.

Two other NMDA inhibitors are dextromethorphan, which is used as a cough suppressant, and ketamine.

Memantine, 10 to 20 mg a day was studied in 28 patients with migraines who were not responding to at least two standard medications. It was found to be effective. A double-blind, placebo-controlled trial of 10 mg of memantine in 52 Iranian patients was also positive. Another double-blind placebo-controlled trial of 60 Indian patients also showed some benefit. A review of case reports and two controlled studies concluded that memantine, 10 to 20 mg a day may be an effective treatment for the prevention of migraines. The only side effects were nausea and dizziness. Overall, memantine is well-tolerated, even in the elderly with Alzheimer's.

I occasionally prescribe memantine and sometimes increase the dose to 20 mg twice a day. I have a few patients who obtained good relief and remain on the drug.

150. Metformin (3)

Metformin (Glucophage, Glumetza) is a drug for the treatment of diabetes and it has not been studied in migraine patients. However, there are several theoretical reasons why it might work.

Obesity does not increase the chance of developing migraines. However, in those who do suffer from migraines an increase in weight is associated with an increase in the frequency and the severity of migraine attacks, according to a study by Drs. Marcelo Bigal, Richard Lipton, and their colleagues. Since metformin is proven to help reduce weight, this could be one of the mechanisms by which it improves migraines. A large 10-year-long study showed that metformin was safe and that weight loss due to metformin was sustainable for up to 10 years.

Another possible mechanism is metformin's direct effect on inflammation, which is one of the major mechanisms involved in migraines. Metformin lowers blood levels of C-reactive protein (CRP). CRP is an inflammatory marker that correlates with the risk of developing chronic migraine.

I prescribe metformin to patients who are overweight. Unlike topiramate, which also helps with weight loss, metformin has few serious side effects. The most common side effect is nausea. Metformin can also cause a drop in vitamin B_{12} level, so a vitamin B_{12} supplement must be taken along with metformin.

I also prescribe metformin to patients with a normal weight if they report having migraines from low blood sugar. This can happen when they are hungry or after eating carbohydrate-rich foods, which can lead to a drop in blood glucose. This is called reactive hypoglycemia. Metformin makes patients feel less hungry and not needing to eat frequently to avoid migraines. Metformin works by regulating the release of glucose from the liver to maintain a steady level of glucose in the blood. It does not cause a drop in blood glucose levels like other diabetes medications. This is why it can be taken by non-diabetics.

Metformin has another potential but unproven benefit – it may make you live longer. For now, it's been shown to be the case only in mice, fruit flies, and worms.

The starting dose of metformin is 500 mg of the long-acting formulation once a day and if necessary, it can be increased to 1,000 and up to 2,000 mg a day.

151. Low-dose naltrexone (2)

Naltrexone is similar to naloxone, a drug used to reverse the effect of an opioid overdose. Naltrexone is mostly used to treat opioid and alcohol dependence and is given as a monthly injection or a daily pill of 50 mg.

Naltrexone blocks the body's endogenous morphine (endorphin) receptors. In theory, this should make the pain worse. However, low-dose naltrexone (LDN). seems to have the opposite effect. A possible explanation is that a small amount of naltrexone blocks the endorphin receptors for a short time, during which the body begins to make more endorphins in an attempt to overcome this block. After the effect of naltrexone wears off, this extra amount of endorphins relieves pain. LDN blocks other receptors (such as Toll-like receptor 4), reduces inflammation, and potentially has other beneficial effects. Most of these effects are not yet proven. Inflammatory bowel diseases such as Crohn's disease and ulcerative colitis do seem to respond to LDN.

A study of 27 patients with chronic central pain syndromes at the Stanford Pain Management Clinic concluded that "The significant findings of decreased average pain scores and depression and improved physical function after prescribing this well-tolerated, inexpensive medication provides justification for larger, controlled trials in patients with central sensitivity syndromes." Some of these central sensitivity syndromes include migraine, fibromyalgia, irritable bowel syndrome, chronic back pain, and others.

Naltrexone is only available in a 50-mg tablet. LDN is started at 1.5 mg nightly for a week, then 3 mg nightly for a week, and then, 4.5 mg nightly. This regimen requires a compounding pharmacy to make capsules containing 1.5 mg for the first two weeks and then, capsules with 4.5 mg. Some of my patients increased the dose to 9 mg nightly. Naltrexone is inexpensive, even considering the cost of compounding.

Because the dose is low, side effects are rare. These include vivid dreams and insomnia. If these side effects occur, the medicine can be taken in the morning.

152. Ketamine (2)

Ketamine (Ketalar) was officially approved for human use by the FDA in 1970. Because of its wide margin of safety, it was administered as a field anesthetic to soldiers during the Vietnam war. Concerns over the psychedelic effects of ketamine and the arrival of new intravenous hypnotics such as propofol led to a marked decrease in the use of ketamine for anesthesia.

In recent years, the use of ketamine has been increasing. Its unique properties have led many researchers to conduct clinical trials for the treatment of pain, depression, and suicidal ideation. Intranasal esketamine (Spravato) is approved by the FDA for treatment-resistant depression.

The degree of efficacy of ketamine for the treatment of pain and migraine headaches is less clear. There have been no double-blind studies of ketamine for the treatment of migraine headaches. There is only anecdotal evidence. A major obstacle to doing such studies is that it is difficult to blind patients to the effect of ketamine on the brain.

A report entitled, Ketamine Infusions for Treatment Refractory Headache describes 77 chronic migraine patients at Thomas Jefferson University who "failed aggressive outpatient and inpatient treatments". These patients were hospitalized and were receiving ketamine infusions for an average of 5 days. Over 70% of these patients improved, although only 27% had sustained improvement.

In another case series published in *The Journal of Headache and Pain,* Drs. Lauritsen, Mazuera, Lipton, and Ashina describe six patients admitted to the hospital with a severe persistent migraine. Their migraines improved with intravenous ketamine, albeit the improvement was only short-term. One patient reported a transient out-of-body hallucination, which resolved after decreasing the rate of infusion.

Intranasal ketamine relieved severe migraine aura in 5 of 11 German patients with familial hemiplegic migraine. In some patients, the aura can be more debilitating than the headache or other symptoms of migraine and we have no effective treatment to stop the aura once it starts.

A study of 18 patients was published in *Neurology* by the headache group at UCSF. It was entitled, *Randomized Controlled Trial of Intranasal Ketamine in Migraine With Prolonged Aura.* It showed that intranasal ketamine reduces the severity but not the duration of migraine aura.

When many more established treatments fail, I do occasionally refer patients for intravenous ketamine infusions. Some of them have found ketamine helpful.

Ketamine is fairly safe since the dose given for pain is much smaller than the dose used for anesthesia. Side effects include sedation, dizziness, dissociation (depersonalization, delusions, hallucinations, feeling cold or hot, and various strange sensations.

153. Methylergonovine (3)

Methylergonovine (Methergine) is used intravenously or in a tablet form after childbirth to help stop bleeding from the uterus. Methylergonovine belongs to the class of drugs known as ergot alkaloids. Dihydroergotamine is a drug in this class that is widely used for the acute treatment of migraines.

Methysergide (Sansert) was another drug in this class. It was effective for the prevention of migraine and cluster headaches. But because of a rare but serious side effect, it was withdrawn from the market. This is unfortunate because for a small group of patients it was the only drug that provided relief. A survey of headache specialists showed that if it was available, the majority would continue to prescribe methysergide to a small number of patients for whom the benefits of improved quality of life outweigh the risks.

After the withdrawal of methysergide, the only oral ergot drug left on the market was methylergonovine. Headache specialists use it for their difficult-to-treat migraine and cluster patients. Methylergonovine was first reported to be effective for the treatment of migraines with medication overuse in an open-label trial of 60 patients in 1993. 44 patients or 73% improved.

Another report by Dr. Loretta Mueller and her colleagues described the effective use of methylergonovine in 20 cluster headache patients.

Intravenous infusion of this drug given to 125 Spanish migraine patients presenting to the emergency room provided pain freedom after one hour in 74%. This was also an uncontrolled, open-label study, which means that the placebo effect probably played a role.

Because methysergide is an ergot alkaloid, we have to assume that its prolonged use also has the potential to cause serious side effects similar to methysergide. This side effect is fibrosis, or the development of scarring around the kidneys, heart, or lungs. Even though it is rare, it is a greatly feared side effect. It can lead to the loss of function in kidneys, heart, or lungs and has no treatment. It is speculated, but not proven, that stopping the drug for a month after 3 or 6 months of continuous use may prevent this side effect.

154. Hydroxyzine (3)

Hydroxyzine (Vistaril) is an old medicine similar to diphenhydramine (Benadryl), cetirizine (Zyrtec), and other anti-histamine drugs. But it has some unique properties. It is the only anti-histamine that is officially approved for "anxiety and tension". It is also approved for itching due to allergic conditions. It is used off-label to treat motion sickness, nausea, vomiting, and dizziness.

Hydroxyzine is often used as an adjuvant analgesic. This means that it can add to pain relief when used with another medication.

A double-blind study compared the injections of 50 mg of hydroxyzine alone, 10 mg of the narcotic nalbuphine (Nubain) alone, a combination of hydroxyzine and nalbuphine, with placebo. It found no benefit from either drug alone or in combination when treating migraines.

A study by the University of Illinois emergency room doctors compared injection of ketorolac with 50 mg of hydroxyzine and 100 mg of meperidine (Demerol, another narcotic). Both treatments had a similar effect. Nausea and drowsiness also occurred at the same rate.

A trial by Dr. Jack Klapper of Denver, CO compared hydroxyzine 75 mg intravenously plus meperidine 75 mg intramuscularly with 1 mg of intravenous DHE plus 10 mg of intravenous metoclopramide (Reglan). Pain reduction was greater with DHE/metoclopramide combination.

There have not been any studies examining the efficacy of oral or injected hydroxyzine alone. It will likely remain an adjuvant or add-on medication for the treatment of migraine headaches.

I sometimes prescribe it to patients whose allergies worsen their migraine headaches or even when there is only a suspicion of an allergic component. It is also useful when anxiety is a contributing factor. For many patients, hydroxyzine is too sedating for daytime use, unless they are treating a severe attack and sedation is an acceptable tradeoff. Most people take 25 or 50 mg nightly, although some tolerate and benefit from 25 mg taken three times a day.

155. Cyproheptadine (2)

Cyproheptadine (Periactin) is one of the most popular drugs for the prevention of migraine headaches in children. There is only one scientific study by Indian doctors suggesting that cyproheptadine (4 mg per day) is as effective as propranolol (80 mg per day) for the prevention of migraines in patients ages 16 to 53. There are no double-blind placebo-controlled trials of this drug in children or adults.

Cyproheptadine is an antihistamine drug, which means that if allergies contribute to migraines, it could help. It is available in 2 mg and 4 mg tablets and the dose ranges from 2 to 12 mg taken at bedtime. Some children can tolerate as much as 8 mg taken three times a day. The drug is popular with pediatricians because it is fairly safe, even if it is not that effective. Common side effects are sleepiness, dizziness, dry mouth, and weight gain.

156. Estrogen/Oral contraceptives (2)

Estrogen can be an effective agent for the treatment of menstrual migraines, according to a report by doctors at The City of London Migraine Clinic. Many women report that their migraines tend to occur before or during their periods and sometimes with ovulation. For some women, menstruation is the only time they get a migraine. The attacks appear to be triggered by a drop in estrogen levels. When estrogen levels stop going up and down as happens during pregnancy and menopause, two out of three women stop having migraines. Although there are many women for whom peri-menopause is when migraines begin.

Continuous contraception means skipping the week of placebo pills. Doing this with an estrogen-containing contraceptive helps maintain a steady level of estrogen. It can prevent the occurrence of periods, menstrual migraines, and other period-related problems such as PMS, painful cramping, and excessive bleeding.

Continuous contraception was first reported in 1970 by doctors at the University of New South Wales to be effective in the prevention of menstrual migraines. Nine out of 22 women had a significant improvement. It is safe to suppress periods for at least a year. Several contraceptives are approved by the FDA for continuous use for 3 months at a time. Low-dose contraceptives such as Lo Loestrin are preferred to those with higher estrogen concentration. The lower the dose of estrogen, the lower the incidence of side effects. In some women, however, this strategy fails and they have breakthrough periods along with breakthrough migraines.

Exogenous estrogen, such as in contraceptives and hormone replacement therapy for menopause, should be avoided in women who have migraines with aura. Estrogen causes a slight increase in the risk of strokes. While this risk is small, if a woman smokes or has other risk factors for strokes, taking estrogen-containing pills is contraindicated. For contraception, such patients can take a progesterone-only pill.

Although one study by Italian researchers reported relief of migraines with a progesterone-only pill in 38 out of 62 women, a review of four such studies suggests only a modest benefit.

157. Opioid drugs (2)

It is not by accident that these drugs are last on my list. The opioid epidemic has been with us for decades. In the 1990s it was fueled in part by the excessive prescribing of opioid drugs. The mistaken belief was that if an opioid is prescribed for the relief of real pain in someone without risk factors for addiction – prior addictions, family history of addictions, criminal record, psychiatric illness – the rate of addiction is extremely low. Now we know that the risk is not so low. Many physicians were disciplined and some even jailed for careless prescribing of opioids. This has led many doctors to stop prescribing opioid drugs altogether.

But an opioid drug can be a life-saver and not a life destroyer for a small and carefully selected group of patients with non-cancer pain, including migraines. In my 30-year career, out of thousands of patients, I've treated only a few dozen with opioid maintenance. The number is so small not only because of my great reluctance to start on this path but also because opioids are not good at relieving migraines.

Doctors with subspecialty training in pain medicine tend to undertake opioid maintenance. I did my pain fellowship from 1984 to 1986 at the Memorial Sloan-Kettering Cancer Center and feel that I can navigate the complexities of this fraught treatment option. I ask every patient to sign an opioid agreement with rules about visits, refills, urine testing, and other precautions.

Methadone, long-acting forms of oxycodone, hydromorphone, and morphine are some of the drugs used for this purpose. Besides addiction, constipation can be a major problem with these drugs. A bowel regimen is started with the first prescription of the opioid drug. This may include a stimulant laxative such as an extract of senna with a stool softener. If constipation is severe, several prescription drugs can help.

Combining drug therapies

Everyone needs to have an abortive drug such as sumatriptan, even if a preventive drug is prescribed. A preventive drug may work very well, but an occasional migraine can still break through. We also sometimes combine two abortive drugs – a triptan with an NSAID or a gepant with an NSAID. As far as preventive medications, when one drug provides partial relief, adding another one of a different class also makes sense. If adding the second drug results in complete relief, you may want to try stopping the first one. Good combinations may be amitriptyline and propranolol, or duloxetine and candesartan. Botox can be combined with any other medication. Drs. Rami Burstein, Messoud Ashina, and their colleagues provide <u>good theoretical reasons to combine Botox with CGRP monoclonal antibodies</u>.

Special circumstances

Menstrual migraine

Most women with menstrual migraines respond well to sumatriptan or another triptan alone or in combination with an NSAID such as ibuprofen or naproxen. If triptans don't work, ubrogepant or rimegepant might.

When these drugs fail, I prescribe mini prophylaxis. This means taking a preventive drug for a week, starting a day or two before the expected migraine attack. Mini prophylaxis can be tried with the usual preventive drugs such as beta-blockers and also with an NSAID or a triptan. Naratriptan and frovatriptan are longer-acting than other triptans but sumatriptan and other short-acting triptans can also prevent migraine attacks.

Continuous contraception can also prevent migraines by preventing periods. This is described in the section on estrogen.

Pregnancy

Two out of three women stop having migraines during pregnancy, especially in the second and third trimester. This is because the estrogen level stops fluctuating. These ups and downs of estrogen are responsible for migraines with menstruation and ovulation.

In some women, however, migraines continue to occur and at times worsen during pregnancy. Most women want to avoid taking any drugs. You can first try to get enough sleep, exercise regularly, maintain a healthy diet, and meditate. In addition to prenatal vitamins, take magnesium.

If medication is unavoidable, sumatriptan or another triptan is a safe choice for abortive therapy. For prevention, Botox is probably the safest and most effective treatment.

Some obstetricians tell women to take acetaminophen or just suffer through their migraines and not take any medicine. I disagree. The distress of having a migraine, especially with vomiting and dehydration is more detrimental to the fetus than taking sumatriptan. Besides being ineffective, acetaminophen may not be as safe as we thought. Children whose mothers took acetaminophen during pregnancy were at about 1.3 times higher risk for ADHD, according to a large Danish study.

Butalbital with caffeine and acetaminophen (Fioricet, Esgic) is another drug prescribed by some obstetricians. They are reassured by its long history of use – about 60 years. Despite its long history, it is only mildly effective and not entirely safe.

Sumatriptan was introduced 20 years ago and the manufacturer has maintained a registry of women who took the drug while pregnant. The final results of this registry were just published in the journal *Headache*. The registry included 626 women who were exposed to sumatriptan during their pregnancies. The risk of major birth defects was not increased.

The authors also reviewed several other large studies that assessed the risk of taking migraine medications during pregnancy. One of the studies was from the Swedish Medical Birth Register, which included 2,257 births following the first-trimester sumatriptan exposure. No risk was found in this study either.

The bottom line is that pregnant women suffering from severe migraines can take sumatriptan. Most women respond to an oral form (tablet), but those with severe attacks should be offered an injection.

If migraines occur for the first time during pregnancy or soon after the delivery, or there is a change in their character, we test for a possible underlying condition. Some of these conditions are thrombosis or an occlusion of a vein in the brain, a drop in thyroid function, or a leak of cerebrospinal fluid.

Neurologists at the Montefiore Headache clinic in the Bronx conducted a 5-year retrospective study of pregnant women who presented with an acute headache, were hospitalized, and received a neurologic consultation.

The researchers identified 140 pregnant women. About 56% of them presented in the third trimester. Primary headaches (migraine and tension-type headaches) were present in 65% and secondary headaches due to underlying disease, 35%. Of the primary headaches, migraine predominated – it was present in 91%. The most common secondary headache disorder was hypertension or high blood pressure. It was found in 51% of women with secondary headaches.

Preeclampsia and eclampsia, a complication of pregnancy, was found in 18%. Pituitary adenoma, a benign tumor, was found in 4%, stroke in 3%, and infection in 2%. Preeclampsia and eclampsia are complications of pregnancy. They consists of increased blood pressure, sometimes seizures, and kidney problems, which can be life-threatening. These conditions are treated with intravenous infusions of large amounts of magnesium.

The authors concluded that among pregnant women receiving inpatient neurologic consultation, more than one-third have secondary headaches. The red flags are the absence of a headache history, presence of hypertension, or fever. Headache features such as the location of pain, throbbing character, sensitivity to light or noise were less helpful in distinguishing primary from secondary headaches. The authors recommend that doctors have a low threshold for doing a CT or MRI scan and stressed the importance of monitoring for preeclampsia and eclampsia.

When nothing works: resistant or refractory migraine

The *European headache federation consensus on the definition of resistant and refractory migraine* was published in 2020:

"*Resistant migraine* is defined by having failed at least 3 classes of migraine preventatives and suffer from at least 8 debilitating headache days per month for at least 3 consecutive months without improvement; definition can be based on review of medical charts. *Refractory migraine* is defined by having failed all of the available preventatives and suffer from at least 8 debilitating headache days per month for at least 6 consecutive months. Drug failure may include lack of efficacy or lack of tolerability. Debilitating headache is defined as a headache causing serious impairment to conduct activities of daily living despite the use of pain-relief drugs with established efficacy at the recommended dose and taken early during the attack; failure of at least two different triptans is required."

The drugs that a patient has to try include injectable CGRP drugs (erenumab, fremanezumab, or galcanezumab), antidepressants (amitriptyline and venlafaxine), antiepileptics (topiramate and valproate), antihypertensives (candesartan and lisinopril, cinnarizine, flunarizine, atenolol, metoprolol, propranolol, or timolol), and Botox.

If a doctor labels you as having refractory migraines, do not despair – these are only 16 out of over 150 methods you can try.

You may also want to examine your life from early childhood for possible emotional, physical, or sexual trauma (see the next section). If you don't feel comfortable discussing this with the doctor or nurse practitioner who is treating your headache, see a mental health professional who specializes in treating trauma.

Post-traumatic stress disorder

Many pain conditions, including migraines, are more likely to occur in people who were abused in childhood. <u>Childhood abuse or neglect was reported by 58% of 1,348 migraine sufferers in a study published in the journal</u> *Headache.* Emotional abuse and neglect were particularly common. Migraine patients who suffered abuse are also more likely to have anxiety and depression.

<u>Another study by Drs. Gretchen Tietjen, Dawn Buse, and their colleagues published in</u> *Neurology* <u>compared the risk of developing migraines with the risk of developing episodic tension-type headache in people who experienced emotional abuse, emotional neglect, or sexual abuse.</u> The incidence of the history of abuse was compared in 8,305 migraine sufferers with that of 1,429 people with tension-type headaches. Episodic tension-type headaches are relatively mild and are experienced by most people. Migraines, on the other hand, are much more severe and often cause an inability to function and interfere with the quality of life.

Emotional neglect and sexual abuse were found to be more common in those with migraines. All three forms of maltreatment were also associated with an increase in migraine headache frequency, but only when anxiety and depression were also present. Only those with emotional abuse had an increased risk of having migraines even if they had no anxiety or depression. This study also showed that having two or three forms of abuse was more likely to cause migraines than if only one type was reported.

Previous studies have also shown a correlation between the number of maltreatment types and pain conditions. These pain conditions include fibromyalgia, irritable bowel syndrome, interstitial cystitis, and temporomandibular joint disorder. Exposure to abuse or a traumatic event may lead to a persistently increased excitability of the nervous system This in turn predisposes one to various pain conditions.

Post-concussion syndrome, which often includes headaches, can persist for many months, especially after minor head trauma. Surprisingly, a mild concussion is more likely to cause a post-concussion syndrome than a severe injury. Little is known, however, about the prognosis after the injury. The symptoms fall into three categories – cognitive (such as memory, concentration difficulties), somatic (headaches, dizziness, etc), and emotional (irritability, anxiety, depression).

A study of 534 patients with a head injury was published by French doctors in *JAMA Psychiatry*. They took into account the fact that injuries are often sustained during psychologically distressing events (car accidents, assaults, falls) and looked for symptoms of post-traumatic stress disorder (PTSD) in those patients.

The authors conducted a study of patients seen at an emergency department for a mild head injury. They checked on these patients for persistent symptoms three months after the concussion. They compared 534 patients with a head injury and 827 control patients with non-head injuries.

The study showed that three months after the injury, 21.2 percent of head-injured and 16.3 percent of nonhead-injured patients had post-concussion syndrome, while 8.8 percent of head-injured patients met the criteria for PTSD compared with only 2.2 percent of control patients.

The doctors concluded that it is important to differentiate post-concussion syndrome from PTSD because it has important consequences, in terms of treatment, insurance resource allocation, and advice provided to patients and their families. They also stressed the importance of considering PTSD in all patients with mild traumatic brain injury who suffer persistent symptoms.

Migraine headaches in patients with PTSD tend to be more frequent and disabling, according to a study of 270 soldiers. Soldiers with PTSD had almost twice as many headaches as soldiers without PTSD. They were more likely to have chronic migraines – headaches occurring on more than 15 days a month. Treatment with preventive medications was less effective in the PTSD group.

Some patients with chronic migraines and pain do not respond to a dozen or more treatments of various types. In many of these patients, the brain has become hyperexcitable due to PTSD. To reduce this hyperexcitability and to relieve chronic migraines requires a combination of medications and specific psychological approaches. Ideally, those with PTSD should be treated by someone who is experienced with this condition. Some of the medications that help PTSD can also have a direct effect on migraines. These are antidepressants, beta-blockers, and epilepsy drugs.

Research studies indicate that having a service dog can also relieve symptoms of PTSD.

Severe PTSD could be part of your migraine problem if you've suffered a traumatic event and have one or both of the following: "feeling upset at reminders" and "avoid thinking or talking about it".

Aura without a headache

While in medical school in my early 20s, I developed my first visual migraine aura without a headache. These auras have continued to occur a few times a year. In my 40s, I started to have migraine headaches without an aura. My auras and headaches continue to happen independently of each other. This is fairly common.

Some patients are bothered by the visual aura more than by the headache which can be mild or even absent. Have your doctor do a blood test to check your level of vitamin B_{12} and a related test, homocysteine, along with RBC magnesium, vitamin D, and other routine tests. People who have migraines with aura or auras without headaches may be more likely to be deficient in vitamin B_{12}. Finding a deficiency is always gratifying because a simple supplement can reduce or stop the attacks.

In some unfortunate patients, the aura can persist for days, weeks, and even months.

A calcium channel blocker, verapamil, and epilepsy drugs, especially lamotrigine, can be helpful. These drugs have not been tested in clinical trials but many headache specialists find them to be effective in some patients.

Migraine with brainstem aura

This condition is better known by its old name, basilar migraine. The term came from the mistaken idea that symptoms result from the constriction of the basilar artery. This artery supplies blood to the brainstem. Symptoms of brainstem dysfunction include dizziness, double vision, unsteadiness, and slurred speech.

Sumatriptan and other triptans are contraindicated in patients with basilar migraine because they are feared to cause worsening of the constriction of blood vessels leading to a stroke. However, now we know that there is no constriction of the basilar artery and that triptans do not cause strokes. We need to educate doctors about replacing the diagnosis of basilar migraine with the diagnosis of migraine with brainstem aura. This will free them to prescribe triptans without fear of causing a stroke.

Hemiplegic migraine

Some patients develop weakness on one side of the body every time they have a migraine. This weakness can occur before the onset of pain and can last 10-60 minutes. At times, the weakness continues into the headache phase and can persist for hours. Hemiplegic migraine often runs in families. Scientists have identified several genetic mutations that are responsible for this condition. Surprisingly, very different genes produce a similar set of symptoms. Some people with hemiplegic migraine have no other family members with this condition. We call this a sporadic form of hemiplegic migraine.

Hemiplegic migraine is a rare condition and it is difficult to gather enough patients for a treatment trial. This means that just like with people who have typical migraines, we keep trying various preventive drugs and hope that one provides relief. I often try verapamil first because several case reports suggest that it works. Acetazolamide, lamotrigine, valproate, and topiramate are some of the other drugs that may help.

Triptans are contraindicated for the acute treatment of hemiplegic migraine. This prohibition is based on an erroneous understanding of what causes weakness. Just like with basilar migraine, in the past, it was logical to think that weakness is due to the lack of blood flow to a part of the brain. And again, because triptans can constrict blood vessels, they were thought to potentially cause a stroke. Now we know that the weakness is caused by the dysfunction of brain cells. Most headache specialists do use triptans to stop attacks of hemiplegic migraine.

Neurologists at the Mayo Clinic reported that Botox injections can relieve not only headache pain, but also associated neurological symptoms, such as visual aura, numbness, and weakness, which can precede or accompany a migraine attack. They describe 11 patients with hemiplegic migraine. Botox was effective in reducing other neurological symptoms, along with headaches, in nine out of 11 patients. Ten of the 11 patients had chronic migraines and on average they did not respond to five preventive drugs before starting Botox.

I have also successfully treated patients with hemiplegic migraines with Botox injections. We have a good understanding of how Botox may relieve pain. It is less clear how it helps neurological symptoms such as weakness, numbness, and visual aura. One theory is that Botox prevents the activation of the peripheral nerves that are needed to generate a migraine attack. This reduces the excitability of the brain and prevents it from generating a migraine attack, including weakness and other symptoms.

Abdominal migraine

According to Oliver Sacks, the best description of abdominal migraine was provided by Edward Liveing in his 1873 book on migraines: "When about 16 years old, enjoying otherwise excellent health, I began to suffer from periodic attacks of severe pain in the stomach ... The seizure would commence at any hour, and I was never able to discover any cause for it, for it was preceded by no dyspeptic symptoms or disordered bowels ... The pain began with a deep, ill-defined uneasiness in the epigastrium. This steadily increased in intensity during the next two or three hours, and then declined. When at its height the pain was very intolerable and sickening—it had no griping quality whatever. It was always accompanied by chilliness, cold extremities, a remarkably slow pulse, and a sense of nausea ... When the pain began to decline there was generally a feeling of movement in the bowels ... The paroxysm left very considerable tenderness of the affected region, which took a day or two to clear off, but there was no tenderness at the time." Years later, this patient ceased to have his abdominal attacks but developed instead attacks of classical migraine coming at similar intervals of three to four weeks.

Out of 1,200 migraine patients he had seen, Oliver Sacks encountered 40 patients who had abdominal attacks similar to those described by Liveing.

As far as treatment of abdominal migraines, sumatriptan and other triptans can be very effective. If attacks are frequent, I try preventive drugs. When none of these drugs work, a few of my patients responded to Botox injections into the skin of the abdomen. It is possible that just like injecting Botox into the scalp reduces sensory input into the brain, injections into the abdominal wall may decrease sensory input from the peripheral nerves in the skin of the abdomen.

Postconcussion migraine

Head injury often leads to headaches and other postconcussion symptoms. In people with a personal or family history of migraines, these headaches usually fit the description of migraines and they are treated as migraines. Trauma can cause a depletion of magnesium and taking a magnesium supplement can help many symptoms. Cognitive-behavioral therapy helps with the psychological trauma that often accompanies a head injury. Botox injections is another effective treatment. Triptans and other acute and preventive medications also help. Eye movement testing and exercises can be very helpful. They are described at the beginning of the book.

Early return to physical and mental activity is more beneficial than complete and prolonged physical and cognitive rest. If you suffered a head injury, try to restart your mental and physical activities as soon as possible. If symptoms worsen, temporarily reduce the intensity, duration, and frequency of these activities.

Vestibular migraine, dizziness, and Mal de Debarquement syndrome

Vestibular migraine has been called migraine-associated vertigo or dizziness and migrainous vertigo. According to the international headache classification, diagnostic criteria include a current or past history of migraine with or without aura, attacks lasting between five minutes and 72 hours, and vestibular symptoms of moderate or severe intensity. The vestibular symptoms include spontaneous vertigo, positional vertigo (vertigo occurring after a change of head position), vertigo triggered by a complex or large moving visual stimulus, head motion-induced vertigo occurring during head motion, and head motion-induced dizziness with nausea. There is also a requirement for at least half of the episodes to be associated with a typical migraine headache or visual aura.

These criteria are the result of a consensus by headache specialists. This means that they are based on the description of cases seen by headache specialists and not large clinical studies. I've encountered some patients who do not have migraine headaches or visual auras but probably suffer from migraine-related dizziness or vertigo. Many migraine sufferers have neck pain and muscle spasm that can also cause or worsen dizziness.

We also lack any studies for the treatment of patients with vestibular migraine. I've often observed that vestibular symptoms improve with the treatment of migraine headaches. In patients who suffer from vestibular symptoms with few or no headaches, I try non-drug migraine treatments first – magnesium, CoQ_{10}, and other supplements, regular aerobic exercise, and meditation.

The international classification of headaches also lists benign paroxysmal vertigo as a condition that occurs in children and which may be associated with migraines. This is different from benign paroxysmal positional vertigo (BPPV) which is triggered by a loose crystal in the inner ear and which can be cured with the Epley maneuver. Migraine-related vertigo usually occurs without a warning and resolves spontaneously after minutes to hours. Patients usually exhibit one of the following features: nystagmus (beating movement of the eyes to one side), unsteadiness, vomiting, paleness, or fearfulness. The neurological examination, audiometry (hearing test) and vestibular function tests are normal between attacks.

Mal de debarquement syndrome (MdDS) or disembarkment syndrome is a rare condition that often, but not always, occurs after getting off a ship. Many people have "sea legs" after getting off a boat but in most people this rocking sensation quickly subsides. Very few unfortunate people continue to have this sensation for months and even years.

One woman told me that she felt that her life was taken away from her. However, despite her symptoms, she was able to hold a full-time job and care for her 3 children. Another patient with a severe case of MdDS had to quit her job and became very anxious and depressed. She never had any anxiety or depression before this illness. This woman also reported feeling tired, being unable to think clearly, having difficulty breathing, having alternating diarrhea and constipation, and other debilitating symptoms.

Almost all patients with MdDS undergo extensive testing, which is usually normal. Vestibular rehabilitation seems to help a few, as does acupuncture, or medications such as clonazepam. Most of the patients with MdDS also suffer from headaches, often migraines.

My experience agrees with a report by a <u>group of doctors from UC Irvine</u> <u>which suggests that treating MdDS as we would vestibular migraine</u> can be effective.

Our research at the New York Headache Center showed that up to 50% of migraine sufferers are deficient in magnesium. This deficiency is not detectable by a routine magnesium test. Other symptoms suggestive of magnesium deficiency include coldness of extremities, or just being cold most of the time, leg or foot muscle cramps (often occurring at night), brain fog or spaciness, difficulty breathing, and other symptoms. Most of the patients with MdDS have many of these symptoms. Many of my patients with MdDS had a dramatic response to an intravenous infusion of magnesium. I often combined it with a vitamin B_{12} injection to correct another common deficiency.

Neck muscle spasm alone can cause a sense of dizziness. In patients with MdDS it makes symptoms worse. Treatment of neck muscle spasm can be of great help.

Cinnarizine or flunarizine (described in the section on preventive drugs) may be worth trying when other measures fail, although these drugs are not available in the US or Canada.

Migraine sufferers are also more likely to have disorders of the inner ear such as BPPV, tinnitus (ringing in the ears), and difficulties with balance and coordination.

New daily persistent headache

New daily persistent headache (NDPH) is one of the dozens of types of headaches listed in the classification of headaches. This particular listing causes more harm than good. NDPH is defined by the single fact that the headache begins on a certain day and persists without a break. The classification says that NDPH may have features suggestive of either migraine or tension-type headache.

There are no parallels to NDPH in medicine. There is no new daily persistent asthma, or new daily persistent colitis, or any other "new daily" disease.

There does not appear to be any justification for having NDPH as a distinct condition. It does not have a typical clinical presentation and it has not led to any research or treatment. When you search for this condition on the internet, you will not find any effective treatment for it. The suffering of many patients is magnified by the loss of hope, worsening depression, and flagging will to live.

Most importantly, some patients with NDPH do respond to treatment. According to anecdotal reports and in my experience, Botox injections, intravenous magnesium, preventive drugs for migraines, and other treatments can be effective.

Status migraine and an emergency room visit

According to the international classification of headaches, a typical migraine attack lasts from 4 to 72 hours. If an attack lasts longer, it is called status migraine. One reason to have the designation of status migraine is to better figure out how to stop a very prolonged attack. Unfortunately, there have not been any scientific studies tackling this problem.

We do have studies of the treatment of severe migraine attacks in the emergency department. They usually do not specify if the attack lasted longer than three days.

Doctors at the emergency room at the Montefiore Hospital in the Bronx conducted a double-blind trial of 330 patients to compare 1) intravenous infusion of 1,000 mg of valproate 2) 10 mg of metoclopramide, and 3) 30 mg of ketorolac. Of patients who received valproate, 69% needed another rescue medication, compared with 33% of those who received metoclopramide and 52% of patients given ketorolac. Sustained headache freedom was achieved by 4% in the valproate group, by 11% in the metoclopramide group, and by 16% receiving ketorolac.

There are not enough headache clinics in the US and other countries, so most people with persistent severe migraines tend to go to an emergency room. Bright lights, noise, and long waits make it the last place you want to be in. It is also hard to think clearly when you are in the throes of a migraine, so you need to be prepared. Have a list of treatments you may want to ask for, just in case the ER doctor is willing to comply with your requests.

If you have been vomiting, first ask for intravenous hydration. Also, ask to have 1 or 2 grams of magnesium added to the intravenous fluids. An injection of sumatriptan can be taken at home and it often eliminates the need to go to an ER. If you don't have it at home, ask for it in the ER. The next best drug is a non-narcotic pain medicine, ketorolac, given intravenously. If you are nauseous, intravenous metoclopramide works well. If these drugs don't help, the next step is intravenous dihydroergotamine. Eight to 12 mg of intravenous dexamethasone can be tried next. In our clinic, besides all these infusions, we also perform nerve blocks and sphenopalatine ganglion blocks. These are rarely done by emergency room doctors.

Headaches often mistaken for migraine

Cluster headaches

There are several similarities between migraine and cluster headaches. Cluster headache is always one-sided. Migraine also often causes pain only on one side of the head. One difference is that cluster headaches occur daily or more than once a day but the duration of an attack is from 30 minutes to 3 hours. Migraine lasts anywhere from 4 to 72 hours. Cluster headaches occur daily for a month or two and then go away for a year or two. Cluster attacks are accompanied by a runny nose or nasal congestion and redness or tearing of the eye on the side of the headache. Nausea, light and noise sensitivity happen rarely with cluster attacks. During a migraine attack, patients prefer to lie down and not move. During a cluster headache, patients become agitated, pace, and sometimes hit their head. Cluster headaches are about five times more common in men while migraines are three times more common in women. This is a relatively rare condition. It strikes about one person in a thousand.

Sumatriptan is approved by the FDA for the acute therapy of cluster and migraine headaches. Galcanezumab is approved for the prevention of both. Oxygen often helps stop a cluster attack but rarely helps migraines. I've had some cluster patients respond well to Botox injections. Epilepsy drugs can help both types of headaches. Verapamil and lithium are effective for the prevention of cluster attacks.

Episodic and chronic paroxysmal hemicrania

The pain always occurs on one side. Attacks occur 5 to 50 times a day with each lasting 2 to 10 minutes. The headache is accompanied by at least two of the following features: redness of the eye, tearing, nasal congestion, runny nose, sweating of the forehead and face, narrowing of the pupil, drooping of the eyelid, and restlessness or agitation.

Paroxysmal hemicranias are indomethacin-sensitive headaches, which means that patients get dramatic relief from indomethacin, one of the strongest NSAIDs. Unfortunately, indomethacin can cause upset stomach, heartburn, and even bleeding ulcers. An herbal supplement boswellia, other NSAIDs and Botox injections sometimes provide good relief.

Hemicrania continua

This headache has similar features to paroxysmal hemicrania but the pain is present continuously. It is also an indomethacin-sensitive headache. Just like with paroxysmal hemicranias, some patients respond to boswellia, other NSAIDs, and Botox injections. Erenumab and other CGRP drugs have helped some of my patients. A single case report also describes a good response to erenumab.

Sinus headaches

Migraines are much more often mistaken for sinus headaches than the other way around. Both can have pain in the area of the frontal (under the forehead) and maxillary (under the cheekbones) sinuses. The pain can be on one side or both. A small amount of clear discharge can occur with migraine headaches. With sinus headaches, the discharge is more copious and is always yellow or green, which is the most telling distinction. Decongestants alone or with aspirin, acetaminophen, or ibuprofen can be effective for milder migraines and sinus headaches. Allergies with nasal congestion or sinus infections can also trigger migraines so they can occur at the same time and may require a specific treatment for each.

Increased cerebrospinal fluid pressure

Headaches from increased cerebrospinal fluid (CSF) pressure has no typical distinguishing features. It can occur weeks and months after a head injury, from certain drugs, a blockage of veins in the brain, infections, and a benign or malignant brain tumor. At times, especially in the early stages, these headaches can resemble migraines. They often cause other neurological and eye findings on the examination. Treatment may include drugs such as acetazolamide and the draining of the fluid through a shunt.

Low cerebrospinal fluid pressure

The headache of low cerebrospinal fluid (CSF) pressure can be very severe. Its main feature is that it quickly gets worse on sitting or standing and just as quickly improves upon lying down. Low CSF pressure often results from the needle going in too far during an epidural steroid injection for low back pain or epidural anesthesia during delivery or surgery. This results in the spinal fluid leaking into the soft tissues of the back. The loss of fluid causes sagging of the brain which normally floats in a thin layer of CSF. Rarely, a spinal fluid leak occurs spontaneously after straining or without an obvious trigger. Spinal fluid leaks can seal on their own but sometimes require a "blood patch"– injecting the patient's blood into the area of the leak. The injected blood clots and seals the leak.

If a CSF leak happens after an epidural procedure, it is better to have the blood patch sooner rather than later. I recommend doing it if the headache persists for more than a couple of days.

Hypnic headaches

These headaches tend to occur after the age of 50 and always wake people from sleep. Migraine can also awake a person from sleep but hypnic headaches tend to last 15 minutes to 3 hours and are not accompanied by other migraine symptoms. Their severity ranges from mild to severe and they can be one-sided. The first simple treatment to try is a cup of coffee before going to bed. Yes, it sounds strange to drink coffee before going to sleep but it seems to work for many people. If caffeine does not help, I try drugs such as lithium and indomethacin.

Dissection of an artery

Dissection of an artery in the neck is a dangerous condition. It can lead to a stroke and even death. In many cases, it can be a benign condition with no lasting ill effects. A study published by German researchers in the journal Cephalalgia indicates that this condition is two times more common in people with migraine headaches. Dissection means that the wall of the artery is split. This can close off blood flow in the artery. In most people, this is not a problem because four arteries in the neck carry blood to the brain. In some, one artery carries a disproportionally large portion of the blood. If that artery gets occluded, the remaining three arteries cannot compensate. This can lead to a stroke. Neurological symptoms suggestive of a stroke include a droopy eyelid, weakness or numbness on one side, difficulty speaking, and others. Neck pain is often the earliest and in benign cases, the only symptom. Because migraine sufferers frequently have neck pain, this complaint is sometimes dismissed as a symptom of migraine. If neck pain is severe and different from the usual neck pain, seek medical attention. The diagnosis is established by an MRA (magnetic resonance angiography) scan.

The increased risk of dissection is one of the reasons to avoid chiropractic adjustments.

Occipital neuralgia

Occipital neuralgia (ON) manifests itself by sharp or electric-like pain in the back of the head. It often occurs on one side but can be bilateral. In addition to pain, some people have numbness or a pins-and-needles sensation in the back of the head. It can occur at any age and may be present in patients who also have migraine headaches. The pain can be worse upon awakening in the morning or after a nap. Sometimes ON begins after a prolonged flight on a plane, after having hair washed at a hairdresser, or following a dental procedure. All these scenarios can lead to the compression of the occipital nerve. Dentists who work for long periods with their head tilted, or secretaries and salespeople who cradle the telephone handset on their shoulder, are susceptible to this condition. In the elderly, arthritic changes in the cervical spine can cause pain, which in turn can cause muscle spasm and entrapment of the occipital nerve. The most effective and quick-acting treatment is a block of the occipital nerve with a local anesthetic, lidocaine. Other effective measures include isometric neck exercises, NSAIDs, tricyclic antidepressants, and Botox injections.

Trigeminal neuralgia

The trigeminal nerve originates from the trigeminal neurons inside the brainstem. Its branches supply sensation to the face and also surround the network of blood vessels that cover the surface of the brain. The trigeminal nerve is intricately involved in the development of migraine headaches. Trigeminal neuralgia (TN) is a very painful condition that has little in common with migraines. The classical form of TN is caused by a compression of one of the two trigeminal nerves by a blood vessel. The symptoms are different from migraine but a few of the features do overlap. This can lead to misdiagnosis. TN causes pain on one side of the face. It can involve one, two, or rarely all three branches of the trigeminal nerve – ophthalmic, maxillary, and mandibular. When the ophthalmic branch is involved it causes pain in the temple and around the eye which can happen with migraines. The pain however is different – it's extremely severe, very brief, and electric-like. A quarter to half of the people with TN has milder continuous pain between the severe bolts. This pain can be throbbing or aching. Occasionally, people feel nauseous from the pain but don't have light or sound sensitivity. They do have a sensitivity to touch but only in a small circumscribed area of the cheek or chin. A light touch or even wind can trigger the electric shock in the face. Chewing, washing face, brushing teeth, and speaking are common triggers. In most patients, pain can be controlled with epilepsy drugs but not the same ones as the ones we use for migraines. A few of my patients with TN have responded well to Botox or erenumab injections.

Sex-induced headache

Headaches that occur during sexual activity tend to elicit fear and embarrassment. Embarrassment is why most people are not aware that this is a fairly common condition. You would not want to share this experience at a party. The fear is justified. A rupture of an aneurysm in the brain can cause a similar severe headache. Fortunately, even though the pain is excruciating, in the vast majority of cases, the pain of a sex-induced headache does not last and does not signify a dangerous problem.

Sex-induced headaches are three times more common in men. In 80% of people, the pain is sudden, occurs at the time of the orgasm, and lasts 30 minutes to a couple of hours. In the remaining 20%, the pain builds up gradually during sex. It often subsides if sexual activity is stopped.

Orgasmic headaches can be recurrent and the pain so severe that some people are afraid to have sex. Sometimes the solution is simple. Take 400 mg of ibuprofen or 500 mg of naproxen an hour before having sex. If this strategy works, after a few times, the medicine can be stopped without a return of headaches. If an over-the-counter medication does not work, a prescription migraine drug, such as sumatriptan can help. Regular exercise can help prevent these headaches in people who are out of shape.

In older people, a common cause of sex-induced headaches is the spasm of neck muscles. These headaches are usually not as intense. Headaches go away if you change the position during sex. They also improve when you strengthen your neck muscles, exercise regularly, and get enough sleep. You can also take ibuprofen before having sex.

Benign exertional headache

Exercise, my number one treatment for migraines, can also cause headaches. The headache can range from mild to excruciating. The pain is usually throbbing in quality, suggesting a connection to migraines. The headache can occur at the start of exercise or only with overexertion. When a severe exertional headache occurs for the first time, an urgent CAT scan of the brain is needed to evaluate for possible bleeding from a ruptured aneurysm. If these headaches persist, an MRI scan may be necessary to look for other brain problems. If we find no underlying cause, treatment begins with physical conditioning. If even mild exertion triggers a headache, ibuprofen or naproxen taken before exercise may prevent the headache. The NSAID needs to be taken only for the first few weeks and then the headaches will often stop occurring.

Tension-type headache

Tension-type headaches are much more common than migraines. However, they rarely impair normal functioning. Doctors sometimes mistake migraines for a tension-type headache. But people with tension-type headaches do well with over-the-counter analgesics and rarely visit doctors. A severe headache is usually a migraine. It is not clear if the term tension refers to mental or muscular tension. Since this is not a disabling condition, little research has been done to figure out the mechanisms leading to tension-type headaches.

The treatment involves all of the general health measures that are recommended in this book for migraine headaches – exercise, sleep, meditation, healthy diet, and others.

Meningitis and other infections

Meningitis headache lacks any specific characteristic but can resemble a severe migraine. Most people also have neck stiffness, fever, and other symptoms. Bacterial meningitis can be a life-threatening emergency and it requires fast treatment. Viral meningitis often occurs with a severe upper respiratory infection that is accompanied by a headache. The only way to differentiate bacterial from viral meningitis is to do a spinal tap.

Other types of infections that can cause severe headaches may occur in immunosuppressed patients. These include tuberculosis, toxoplasmosis, and cryptococcus. An otherwise healthy patient who came to the US from Russia a few years earlier presented to me with 6 months of severe migraine-like headaches. An MRI scan of her brain was consistent with chronic meningitis. I did a spinal tap that revealed tuberculous meningitis.

Patients often ask me about the possibility of Lyme disease causing their headaches. It is unusual for Lyme disease to cause headaches and no other symptoms.

Brain tumor headache

Brain tumor headaches can mimic migraines. However, it is unlikely that a malignant brain tumor will cause headaches for a long time without any additional neurological symptoms. These may include difficulty with speech, vision, weakness or numbness on one side, or seizures. If the tumor is benign (most commonly a meningioma or pituitary adenoma), it can cause headaches of long duration and additional symptoms can take a long time to develop. These headaches rarely present as a typical migraine and usually lead to an investigation with a CT or MRI scan.

Migraine drugs such as sumatriptan should not work for a brain tumor headache, but at times they do. Headaches due to a brain tumor or an aneurysm rupture can respond to sumatriptan. Botox can also help brain tumor headaches. So just because a migraine drug stops a headache, it does not mean that the headache is a migraine.

Aneurysm headache

When someone says, I have the worst headache of my life, doctors are taught to think of a ruptured brain aneurysm. An aneurysm is an outpouching of an artery in the brain. This sac has thin walls and is more likely to rupture as it gets bigger. The risk of rupture is low if the aneurysm is smaller than 5 mm. The size is established by an angiogram. Usually, it causes one big headache when it ruptures. Unfortunately, 40% of people die before they reach the hospital. In a small percentage of people, the aneurysm does not rupture but has a small leak causing a milder headache. These are called sentinel headaches and they allow for the timely diagnosis and treatment of the aneurysm.

Aneurysms sometimes run in the family. If you have a first-degree relative who had a brain aneurysm, it is worth having an MRA.

Stroke headaches

About 40% of people with strokes due to an occlusion of an artery have a headache at the time of the stroke. When the stroke is due to bleeding, headache is almost always present. Strokes rarely present only with a headache and without any other neurological signs and symptoms.

Exploding head syndrome

This condition is not a headache since the person does not have any pain, but it is often reported as a headache. It always wakes a patient from sleep and they feel like an explosion went off in their head. At times they see a flash of light. The sensation is momentary but frightening. Most people can go back to sleep. Attacks tend to be infrequent and do not require treatment.

Headache due to drugs

Medication-induced headaches are extremely common. They can resemble migraines, can occur from almost any drug, and usually are easy to diagnose. At times, the link is not obvious because the headaches occur gradually. Drugs that most often cause headaches are oral contraceptives, other forms of estrogen, acid reflux drugs called proton pump inhibitors (omeprazole and others), antihistamines called H-2 blockers (ranitidine and similar drugs), certain asthma medications such as albuterol, antidepressants, drugs for erectile dysfunction, stimulants, and blood pressure medications. Note that some of the same drugs that are used to treat headaches can cause or worsen them.

Temporal arteritis

Temporal arteritis is an inflammation of the arteries around the brain and scalp. It occurs in one out of 5,000 people over 50. Women are three to four times more likely to be affected. It rarely happens in people younger than 60. It becomes more common with advancing age. Temporal arteritis is also called giant cell arteritis because giant cells can be seen under the microscope in the arteries.

Headache is often the first symptom and the pain is typically felt in one temple, mimicking a migraine. The headache can also involve other parts of the head and occur on both sides. If left undiagnosed and untreated, temporal arteritis can cause a stroke and blindness in one or both eyes.

Besides headaches, temporal arteritis can cause neck and jaw pain, general weakness, muscle aches, and a mild fever. The preliminary diagnosis is established by blood tests. It can be confirmed by a biopsy of the temporal artery. Polymyalgia rheumatica is a related rheumatological condition that causes severe muscle pains. It can occur alone or with temporal arteritis.

Temporal arteritis and polymyalgia rheumatica are treated with steroid medications, such as prednisone. Since migraine can also respond to prednisone, this is not a differentiating factor.

Glaucoma headache

Glaucoma is an eye disease that is caused by increased pressure inside the eye. It usually develops gradually and causes visual problems first. If it starts suddenly, it can mimic a migraine attack. Acute-closure glaucoma causes a severe headache, nausea, vomiting, and blurred vision – all typical symptoms of a migraine.

My top 10 migraine treatments

Non-drug therapies

1. Aerobic exercise

2. Meditation

3. Magnesium

4. CoQ10

Abortive drugs

1. Sumatriptan

2. Rimegepant

3. Naproxen

Preventive drugs

1. Botox

2. Galcanezumab

3. Nebivolol

Please read this notice

The advice in this book is not intended to replace treatment by a medical professional. I hope it will educate you and make you better prepared when you do see a doctor or a nurse practitioner.

About the Author

A lexander Mauskop, MD, is the Director and founder of the New York Headache Center in New York City. He is Board-certified in Neurology with subspecialty certification in Headache Medicine. Dr. Mauskop is a Fellow of the American Academy of Neurology and the American Headache Society. He is a Professor of Clinical Neurology at SUNY, Downstate Medical Center.

Dr. Mauskop has conducted breakthrough research in the field of headaches and has published numerous articles in scientific journals. He serves as a reviewer for *The New England Journal of Medicine, Neurology, Headache*, and other medical journals. In addition to having given over 500 lectures, he has been a guest speaker at Cornell, Harvard, Columbia, NYU and Dartmouth Medical Schools, Mayo and Cleveland Clinics, as well as Charité – Universitätsmedizin Berlin, Europe's largest university hospital, and Ludwig-Maximilians-Universität München.

Dr. Mauskop has organized and directed an annual educational symposium for physicians in New York City for 25 years. Over 200 doctors from around the world have visited the New York Headache Center to learn advanced treatment techniques, including Botox injections, magnesium infusions, and others. Two editions of his book for doctors, *Migraine and Headache* have been published by Oxford University Press. He is also the author of *The Headache Alternative: A Neurologist's Guide to Drug-Free Relief,* a book published by Dell, and *What Your Doctor May Not Tell You About Migraines: The Breakthrough Program That Can Help End Your Pain*, published by Warner Books.

You can read about the latest developments in the field of headaches on Dr. Mauskop's blog – nyheadache.com/blog. The blog has had over a million visitors.

Made in the USA
Coppell, TX
22 June 2021

57931102R00105